ALLE ZEIT WACH
SJ
1842

New Aspects of the Role of Adrenoceptors in the Cardiovascular System

Festschrift in honour of the 65th birthday of Prof. Dr. Hans-Joachim Schümann

Edited by
Horst Grobecker   Athineos Philippu   Klaus Starke

With 76 Figures and 13 Tables

Springer-Verlag Berlin Heidelberg New York
London Paris Tokyo

Professor Dr. med. Horst Grobecker
Lehrstuhl für Pharmakologie, Universität Regensburg
Universitätsstraße 31, 8400 Regensburg
Federal Republic of Germany

Professor Dr. med. Athineos Philippu
Institut für Pharmakodynamik und Toxikologie, Universität Innsbruck
Peter-Mayr-Straße 1, 6020 Innsbruck
Austria

Professor Dr. med. Klaus Starke
Pharmakologisches Institut, Universität Freiburg
Hermann-Herder-Straße 5, 7800 Freiburg i. Br.
Federal Republic of Germany

The symposion has made been possible by generous support from the following sponsors:
Astra Chemicals, Wedel Holstein
Bayer AG, Leverkusen
Boehringer Ingelheim, Ingelheim
Boehringer Mannheim GmbH, Mannheim
Hoechst AG, Frankfurt a. M.
Klinge-Pharma GmbH & Co., München
Pfizer GmbH, Karlsruhe
Sandoz AG, Nürnberg
Sanol Schwarz GmbH, Monheim

The editors acknowledge this support and would like to thank Dr. T. Kreuzer and his coworkers from Astra Chemicals for the excellent local organisation.

ISBN-13: 978-3-642-71315-6 e-ISBN-13: 978-3-642-71313-2
DOI: 10.100/978-3-642-71313-2

Library of Congress Cataloging in Publication Data
New aspects of the role of adrenoceptors in the cardiovascular system. Based on a symposium held on Feb. 14-16, 1985 in Hamburg in honor of the 65th birthday of Professor Hans-Joachim Schümann. Bibliography: p. Includes index.
1. Adrenergic receptors--Congresses. 2. Cardiovascular system--Congresses. I. Grobecker, H. (Horst), 1934-. II. Philippu, A. (Athineos), 1931-. III. Starke, K. (Klaus), 1937-. IV. Schümann, Hans-Joachim.
QP110.A37N48 1986 612.1 86-10216

Softcover reprint of the hardcover 1st edition 1986

Typesetting and Bookbinding: Appl, Wemding; Printing: aprinta Wemding
2127/3145-5 4 3 2 1 0

Preface

This volume is the product of a symposium held on 14–16 February, 1985 in Hamburg in honour of the 65th birthday of Prof. Hans-Joachim Schümann.

Schümann was born on 28 December, 1919 in Stralsund. He studied medicine in Cologne, Greifswald and Rostock. The chair of pharmacology in Rostock was held at that time by Peter Holtz. It was he who first introduced Schümann to pharmacology in 1944 and who was his *Doktorvater* (research supervisor). After the war, Schümann again worked with Holtz in Rostock and then in Frankfurt am Main. He received decisive stimuli during a research fellowship, in 1956, in Prof. J. H. Burn's department in Oxford, where he also worked with Prof. H. Blaschko. In 1964 he accepted his present position as *ordentlicher* (full) *Professor* and Head of the Institute of Pharmacology and Toxicology of the then newly founded Medical Faculty of Essen. He has remained in Essen despite being offered the chair of pharmacology in Göttingen in 1968.

It is interesting to observe how in the main lines of his scientific work, which now spans 40 years, Schümann has followed the steps involved in autonomic neurotransmission from transmitter release to transmitter-receptor interaction. He started with the identification of noradrenaline as an adrenal medullary hormone in its own right; continued with research on the vesicular storage of catecholamines, including the co-storage of catecholamines and ATP; then studied the presynaptic modulation of the release of noradrenaline; and in the last few years has concentrated on postsynaptic catecholamine receptors; in this field, his thorough investigations on myocardial α-adrenoceptors are particularly noteworthy.

Schümann was President of the German Pharmacological Society from 1971 to 1974. He was elected an Affiliate Member of the Royal Society of Medicine (London) and is also an Honorary Member of the Japanese Pharmacological Society.

In Hamburg, his students, co-workers and colleagues from six countries joined Jochen and Annelies Schümann to celebrate a careful and stimulating scientist and a faithful and warm friend. The scientific papers read at the symposium and printed here reflect much of Schümann's own work as outlined above: from the central nervous control of blood pressure, via the mechanism and possible physiological function of the presynaptic modulation of sympathetic transmitter release, to myocardial and vascular adrenoceptors. May the volume express the contributors' esteem for a teacher, colleague and friend.

The editors

Table of Contents

List of Contributors

Brodde, O.-E., Professor Dr.
Abteilung für Nieren- und Hochdruckkranke, Nephrologisches Labor, Medizinische Klinik und Poliklinik, Universitätsklinikum Essen, Hufelandstraße 55, 4300 Essen 1, Federal Republic of Germany

Endoh, M., Professor Dr.
Department of Pharmacology, Yamagata University School of Medicine, Nishinomae, Zao-iida, 990-23 Yamagata, Japan

Ensinger, H., Dr.
Pharmakologisches Institut, Universität Freiburg, Hermann-Herder-Straße 5, 7800 Freiburg i. Br., Federal Republic of Germany

Göthert, M., Professor Dr.
Institut für Pharmakologie und Toxikologie, Universität Bonn, Reuterstraße 2b, 5300 Bonn 1, Federal Republic of Germany

Grobecker, H., Professor Dr.
Lehrstuhl für Pharmakologie, Universität Regensburg, Universitätsstraße 31, 8400 Regensburg, Federal Republic of Germany

Groß, G., Privat-Dozent Dr.
Pharmakologisches Institut, Universitätsklinikum Essen, Hufelandstraße 55, 4300 Essen 1, Federal Republic of Germany

Guimarães, S., Professor Dr.
Department of Pharmacology, Medical Faculty, 4200 Porto, Portugal

Hedler, L., Dr.
Pharmakologisches Institut, Universität Freiburg, Hermann-Herder-Straße 5, 7800 Freiburg i. Br., Federal Republic of Germany

Hentrich, F., Privat-Dozent Dr.
Pharmakologisches Institut, Universitätsklinikum Essen, Hufelandstraße 55, 4300 Essen 1, Federal Republic of Germany

Majewski, H., Dr.
Department of Pharmacology, University of Melbourne, Parkville, Victoria 3052, Australia

Nedergaard, O. A., Professor Dr.
Department of Pharmacology, Odense University School of Medicine, J. B. Winsløws Vej 19, 5000 Odense C, Denmark

Osswald, W., Professor Dr.
Department of Pharmacology, Faculty of Medicine, 4200 Porto, Portugal

Philippu, A., Professor Dr.
Institut für Pharmakodynamik und Toxikologie, Universität Innsbruck, Peter-Mayr-Straße 1, 6020 Innsbruck, Austria

Rodrigues-Pereira, E., Professor Dr.
Department of Pharmacology, Faculty of Medicine, 4200 Porto, Portugal

Scholz, H., Professor Dr.
Abteilung Allgemeine Pharmakologie, Universitäts-Krankenhaus Eppendorf, Martinistraße 52, 2000 Hamburg 20, Federal Republic of Germany

Starke, K., Professor Dr.
Pharmakologisches Institut, Universität Freiburg, Hermann-Herder-Straße 5, 7800 Freiburg i. Br., Federal Republic of Germany

Stjärne, L. Professor Dr.
Department of Physiology, Karolinska Institutet, 10401 Stockholm, Sweden

Szabo, B., Dr.
Pharmakologisches Institut, Universität Freiburg, Hermann-Herder-Straße 5, 7800 Freiburg i. Br., Federal Republic of Germany

I. Neuronal Adrenoceptors in Cardiovascular Regulation

Involvement of Catecholaminergic Neurones of the Hypothalamus in Blood Pressure Regulation

A. Philippu

Institut für Pharmakodynamik und Toxikologie, Universität Innsbruck Peter-Mayr-Straße 1, 6020 Innsbruck, Austria

One of the criteria for the involvement of a brain neurotransmitter in blood pressure regulation is the influence of blood pressure changes on the release of the neurotransmitter. If the transmitter were indeed involved in the homeostasis of blood pressure, then changes in blood pressure would be expected to modify the rate of transmitter release in brain areas involved in cardiovascular control, thus counteracting the blood pressure change.

The involvement of catecholaminergic neurones of the hypothalamus in blood pressure regulation was investigated by using push-pull cannulae inserted into the posterior and/or anterior hypothalamic areas of anaesthetized and conscious, freely moving animals. The hypothalamic areas were superfused with artificial cerebrospinal fluid (CSF) through the push-pull cannulae. The release of endogenous catecholamines was radioenzymatically determined in the superfusates under resting conditions, as well as during experimentally induced blood pressure changes. Furthermore, the feedback regulation of the catecholamine release was studied by superfusion of the cat hypothalamus with CSF which contained agonists and antagonists of α- and β-adrenoceptors. Finally, the posterior or anterior hypothalamic areas were superfused through push-pull cannulae and electrically stimulated with the non-insulated tips of the cannulae. The effects of alpha- or beta-adrenoceptor agonists and antagonists on the stimulation-induced blood pressure changes were investigated.

Resting Release of Catecholamines

The resting catecholamine release pattern was studied in the posterior hypothalamic area of the anaesthetized cat and in the posterior and anterior hypothalamic areas of the conscious rabbit. In both animal species, the rates of dopamine, noradrenaline, and adrenaline release varied rhythmically with time. In the posterior hypothalamus of the cat (Fig. 1), the rates of amine release varied with a frequency of one cycle per 70 min. In the posterior and anterior hypothalamic areas of the rabbit (Fig. 2), the ultradian rhythm had a frequency of 64 and 74 min respectively. Thus, in the hypothalamus of anaesthetized and conscious animals, the rates catecholamine release follow an ultradian rhythm with a periodicity of approximately 70 min (Philippu et al. 1979; Robinson et al. 1983). In this connection, it is noteworthy that the plasma noradrenaline level also shows an ultradian rhythm with a cycle duration of 90 min (Levin et al. 1978). It is likely that the periodicity in the plasma

New Aspects of the Role of Adrenoceptors in the
Cardiovascular System/Ed. by Grobecker et al.

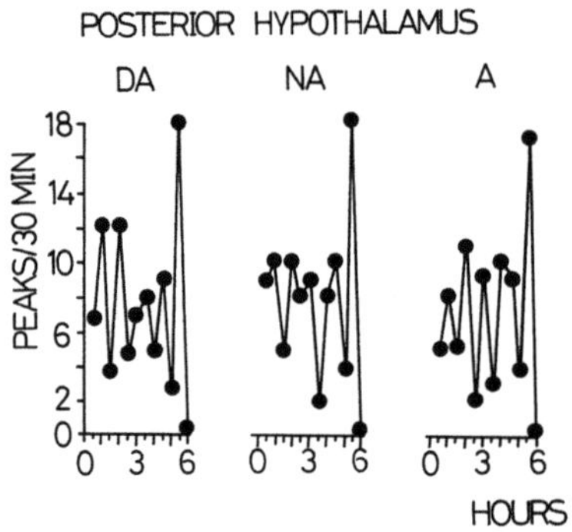

Fig. 1. Resting release of catecholamines in the posterior hypothalamus of anaesthetized cats. The superfusate was continuously collected in 15 min periods. Frequency polygons were drawn by plotting number of peaks of high rates of release per 30 min against time. *DA* dopamine, *NA* noradrenaline, *A* adrenaline. Mean values of 16 experiments. Modified from Philippu et al. (1979)

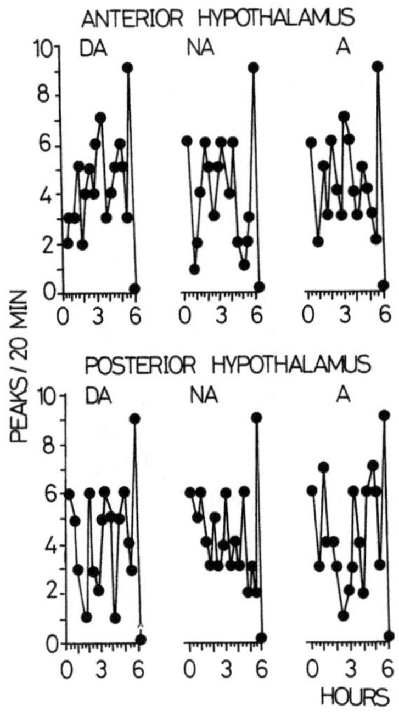

Fig. 2. Resting release of catecholamines in the anterior and posterior hypothalamus of conscious rabbits. The superfusate was continuously collected in 10 min periods. Frequency polygons were drawn by plotting number of peaks of high rates of release per 30 min against time. *DA* dopamine, *NA* noradrenaline, *A* adrenaline. Mean values of 9 experiments. Modified from Robinson et al. (1983)

level of noradrenaline, as well as periodicities in the functions of peripheral organs innervated by the vegetative system, are dependent on the rhythmic release of neurotransmitters in the hypothalamus. A similar rhythmic release of endogenous catecholamines was recently observed in the nucleus tractus solitarii of anaesthetized cats (Lanzinger et al. 1986).

Feedback Regulation of Catecholamine Release

Transection of the brain caudal to the hypothalamus abolishes the release of the three catecholamines in the posterior hypothalamus of the anaesthetized cat and strongly reduces the release in the anterior hypothalamic area. In this area, catecholamine release is abolished after circular transection around the hypothalamus. Hence, the catecholamine release in the posterior hypothalamus is dependent on impulses which generate in the catecholaminergic cell bodies localized in the brain stem, while the catecholaminergic nerve endings of the anterior hypothalamus seem to partly originate from cell bodies localized lateral or rostral to the hypothalamus (Dietl et al. 1981 b). These findings show that under in vivo conditions, the so-called resting release of catecholamines in the hypothalamus is actually a stimulus-induced release.

The stimulus-induced release was used to investigate the presynaptic regulation of the catecholamine release in the brain under in vivo conditions. For this purpose, the posterior hypothalamic area of the anaesthetized cat was continuously superfused with CSF and the superfusate was collected in 15-min intervals. The hypothalamus was superfused with drug-containing CSF for 15 min. Superfusion with the α-adrenoceptor blocking agent yohimbine (10 µmol/liter) enhanced the rates of release of all three catecholamines. The effect of yohimbine was abolished after brain transection caudal to the hypothalamus, thus showing the stimulus-dependence of the drug effect (Fig. 3).

Superfusion with the β_1- and β_2-adrenoceptor agonist isoprenaline (50 µmol/liter) greatly enhanced the release of the catecholamines, while superfusion with the non-selective β-adrenoceptor blocking agent propranolol reduced their rates of release. Since the β_1-agonist tazolol and the β_2-agonist salbutamol enhanced the rates

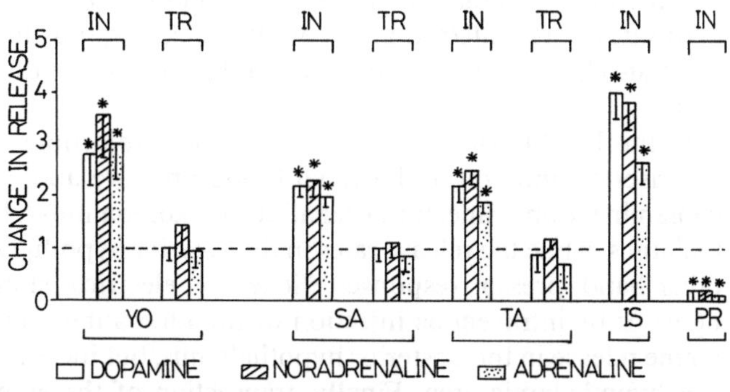

Fig. 3. Effect of superfusion of the posterior hypothalamus of the anaesthetized cat with drugs affecting adrenoceptors on the release of catecholamines. The rates of release of the catecholamines before superfusion with drugs were taken as 1.0. The superfusate was continuously collected in 15 min periods. *IN* release of catecholamines in animals with intact brain, *TR* release in animals after transection of the brain caudal to the hypothalamus. *YO* yohimbine (10^{-5} mol/liter), *SA* salbutamol (5×10^{-5} mol/liter), *TA* tazolol (5×10^{-5} mol/liter), *IS* isoprenaline (5×10^{-5} mol/liter), *PR* propranolol (5×10^{-5} mol/liter). Mean values of 4-12 experiments ± S.E.M. Asterisks denote statistical significance between rate of release in the sample preceeding superfusion with drug and that on superfusion with drug-containing CSF. $^*P < 0.05$. Modified from Dietl et al. (1981 a)

of release, β_1- and β_2-adrenoceptors seem to be involved in the feedback regulation of catecholamine release. The effects of these drugs were also abolished after transection of the brain caudal to the hypothalamus (Fig. 3). Thus, under in vivo conditions, the release of catecholamines is modulated by a negative feedback mechanism (via α_2-receptors) and by a positive feedback mechanism (via β_1- and β_2-receptors; Dietl et al. 1981 a).

The results obtained with the β-agonists and propranolol correspond to the observation that tazolol, salbutamol and isoprenaline facilitate, while propranolol reduces the release of endogenous dopamine from slices of rat brain (Ueda et al. 1983, 1984). It has been suggested that adrenaline activates prejunctional β-adrenoceptors at sympathetic nerve endings, thus leading to an increased release of noradrenaline (for review see Majewski 1983). It is likely that hypothalamic superfusion with β-agonists or antagonists alters the rate of adrenaline release. This in turn modulates the rates of release of the other catecholamines by acting on β-receptors located at noradrenergic and dopaminergic nerve endings. Experimentation with extremely short collection periods of the superfusate (1- to 10-s collection periods) may help in investigating whether a sequential release of the catecholamines indeed exists.

Changes in Blood Pressure Alter the Rates of Catecholamine Release

Several procedures were introduced in order to induce blood pressure changes experimentally: (1) Drugs that either increase or decrease arterial blood pressure were injected intravenously. (2) Controlled bleeding was induced. (3) The peripheral trunk of the dissected splanchnic nerve was electrically stimulated. (4) The spinal cord was transected between C1 and C2. In most of these experiments, superfusates were collected at 90- or 10-s intervals, thus making it possible to closely correlate changes in blood pressure and alterations in the rates of catecholamine release.

Controlled bleeding as well as intravenous injections of sodium nitroprusside or chlorisondamine lowered arterial blood pressure and enhanced the rates of catecholamine (dopamine, noradrenaline and adrenaline) release in the posterior hypothalamus, while the release rates in the anterior hypothalamus were reduced. On the other hand, pressor responses elicited by electrical stimulation of the splanchnic nerve or by intravenous injection of noradrenaline reduced the rates of catecholamine release in the posterior hypothalamus, but increased their release in the anterior hypothalamic area. Finally, transection of the spinal cord led to a biphasic change in blood pressure. A short pressor response was followed by a long period of hypotension. The pressor response, which was probably due to mechanical stimulation of descending pathways, was associated with a decreased release of catecholamines in the posterior hypothalamus and an increased release in the anterior hypothalamus. The hypotensive phase, a result of the interruption of blood vessel innervation, enhanced catecholamine release in the posterior hypothalamus, but decreased the rate of release in the anterior hypothalamus (Table 1).

Table 1. Effects of experimentally induced blood pressure changes on the release of endogenous catecholamines in the posterior and anterior hypothalamic areas

Change in Blood Pressure	Rates of Release of Dopamine, Noradrenaline and Adrenaline	
	Posterior Hypothalamus	Anterior Hypothalamus
Fall	Increase	Decrease
Rise	Decrease	Increase

The time courses of the blood pressure changes coincided fairly well with the changes in catecholamine release. The changes in the catecholamine release rate were much more pronounced in conscious animals than in anaesthetized animals, which indicates that pentobarbital anaesthesia reduces the responsiveness of catecholaminergic neurones in the hypothalamus to blood pressure changes. This corresponds to the observation that the drug dosage required to affect arterial pressure is higher in conscious animals than in anaesthetized animals (Sinha et al. 1980; Philippu et al. 1980; Dietl et al. 1981a; Philippu et al. 1981; Robinson et al. 1983).

Therefore, changes in arterial blood pressure affect the rates of catecholamine release oppositely in the two hypothalamic areas. These findings indicate that catecholaminergic neurones of the hypothalamus are involved in the homeostasis of the arterial blood pressure.

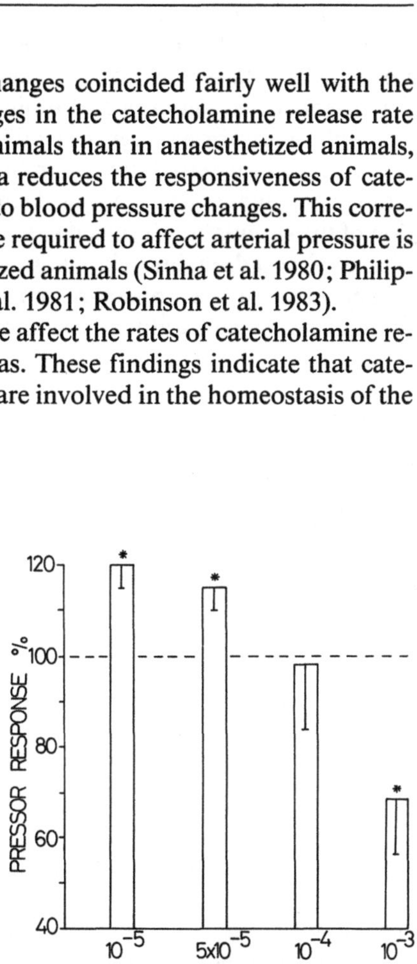

Fig. 4. Effect of superfusion of the posterior hypothalamus of the anaesthetized cat with various concentrations of clonidine on the pressor response to hypothalamic stimulation. The posterior hypothalamus was electrically stimulated every 10 min before and on hypothalamic superfusion with drugs. Superfusion with drugs lasted for 60 min. Shown are changes in the pressor response 60 min after beginning the superfusion with clonidine-containing CSF. The pressor response before starting superfusion with the drug was taken as 100%. For statistical analysis the pressor responses were compared with those obtained in control animals, in which the posterior hypothalamus was superfused with drug-free CSF. Mean values of 6 experiments ± S.E.M. *$P<0.05$. Modified from Philippu et al. (1974)

Hypothalamic superfusion with drugs influences the blood pressure changes elicited by electrical stimulation of the superfused area

It seems likely that the released catecholamines stimulate adrenoceptors located on catecholaminergic or noncatecholaminergic neurons of the hypothalamus, thus counteracting the experimentally induced blood pressure changes. The involvement of adrenoceptors in the cardiovascular responses to centrally released catecholamines has been investigated in anaesthetized cats. Electrical stimulation of the posterior hypothalamus with the non-insulated tip of the push-pull cannula led to a rise in blood pressure which was enhanced on hypothalamic superfusion with alpha-adrenoceptor agonists and inhibited when the hypothalamus was superfused with alpha-receptor antagonists (Philippu et al. 1973, 1974). Low concentrations of clonidine also increased the rise in blood pressure elicited by hypothalamic stimulation, while high concentrations decreased the pressor response (Fig. 4). The inhibition of the stimulation-induced rise in blood pressure was attributed to a decreased release of noradrenaline via stimulation of presynaptic alpha-adrenoceptors, the enhancement of the pressor response by low clonidine concentrations to stimulation of postsynaptic alpha-receptors (Philippu et al. 1974). The increase by cloni-

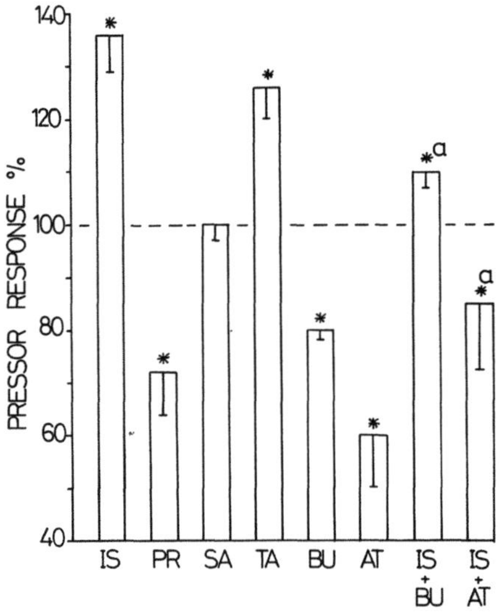

Fig. 5. Effect of superfusion of the posterior hypothalamus of the anaesthetized cat with β-receptor agonists or antagonists on the pressor response to hypothalamic stimulation. The posterior hypothalamus was electrically stimulated every 10 min before and on hypothalamic superfusion with drugs. Superfusion with drugs lasted for 60 min. Drug concentrations: *IS* isoprenaline, *PR* (±)-propranolol, *SA* salbutamol, *BU* butoxamine, *AT* atenolol: 10^{-3} mol/liter, *TA* taxolol: 5×10^{-4} mol/liter. Shown are changes in the pressor responses 60 min after beginning the superfusion with drug-containing CSF. The pressor response before starting superfusion with drugs was taken as 100%. For statistical analysis the pressor responses were compared with those obtained in control animals, in which the posterior hypothalamus was superfused with drug-free CSF. Mean values of 5–6 experiments ± S.E.M. *$P < 0.05$, *a denotes statistical significance between superfusion with isoprenaline and superfusion with isoprenaline in the presence of a β-receptor antagonist. Modified from Philippu and Stroehl (1978)

dine of the pressor response is in accordance with the observation that in conscious animals central administration of clonidine increases blood pressure by acting on bulbar and suprabulbar adrenoceptors (Trolin 1975; Correa et al. 1982; Vlahakos et al. 1985; Kawasaki and Takasaki 1986).

Hypothalamic superfusion with beta-adrenoceptor blocking drugs decreased the pressor response, while superfusion of the hypothalamus with the beta-receptor agonists orciprenaline or isoprenaline enhanced the pressor response to hypothalamic stimulation (Philippu and Kittel 1977; Philippu and Stroehl 1978). To characterize the type of beta-adrenoceptors involved in the pressor response, the hypothalamus was superfused with selective agonists and antagonists of beta-receptors. The selective $beta_2$-receptor agonists salbutamol and terbutaline were ineffective, while the selective $beta_1$-agonist tazolol enhanced the pressor response (Fig. 5), thus indicating the involvement of $beta_1$-receptors in the rise in blood pressure elicited by hypothalamic stimulation. As it might be expected, hypothalamic superfusion with the $beta_1$-receptor antagonist atenolol greatly inhibited the pressor response. Moreover, superfusion with atenolol abolished and even slightly reversed the effect of isoprenaline on the pressor response. Butoxamine, which selectively blocks $beta_2$-receptors, also reduced the pressor response and inhibited the effect of isoprenaline, but these

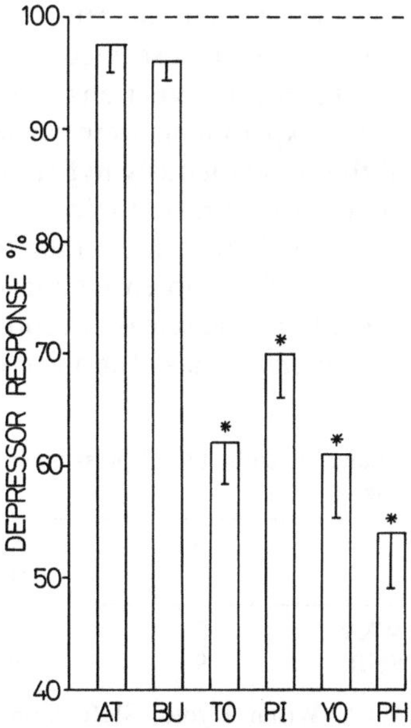

Fig. 6. Effect of superfusion of the anterior hypothalamus of the anaesthetized cat with alpha- or beta-receptor antagonists on the depressor response to hypothalamic stimulation. The anterior hypothalamus was electrically stimulated every 10 min before and on hypothalamic superfusion with drugs. Superfusion with drugs lasted for 60 min. Drug concentrations: atenolol, butoxamine: 10^{-3} mol/liter, tolazoline, piperoxan, yohimbine, phentolamine: 10^{-4} mol/liter. Shown are changes in the depressor responses 60 min after beginning the superfusion with drug-containing CSF. For statistical analysis the pressor responses were compared with those obtained in control animals, in which the anterior hypothalamus was superfused with drug-free CSF. Mean values of 6 experiments ± S.E.M. $^{*}P < 0.05$. Modified from Philippu and Schartner (1976) and Iijima and Philippu (1980)

inhibitory effects of butoxamine were less pronounced than those observed with atenolol (Philippu and Stroehl 1978). It seems that predominantly beta$_1$-receptors of the posterior hypothalamus are involved in the pressor response to hypothalamic stimulation.

Electrical stimulation of the anterior hypothalamus decreases blood pressure. Superfusion of this hypothalamic area with alpha-adrenoceptor blocking agents antagonized the depressor response, while beta-receptor antagonists were ineffective (Philippu and Schartner 1976; Iijima and Philippu 1980) (Fig. 6).

These results suggest that hypothalamic stimulation releases locally catecholamines which stimulate beta- and/or alpha-adrenoceptors, thus leading to blood pressure changes. Similarly, experimentally induced blood pressure changes (see above) seem to alter the rates of catecholamine release from the hypothalamic nerve terminals so as to counteract the blood pressure change.

Release of Catecholamines in Normotensive and Spontaneously Hypertensive Rats

Since catecholamine release in the hypothalamus was dependent on the arterial blood pressure, it seemed of interest to study amine release in the hypothalamus of spontaneously hypertensive rats.

The experiments were carried out in 60-day-old rats. The systolic arterial pressure of the spontaneously hypertensive rats was 29 mm Hg higher than in normotensive Wistar Kyoto rats (Table 1). In the posterior nucleus of the hypothalamus of spontaneously hypertensive rats the rate of release of dopamine was higher than in the nucleus of normotensive rats (Fig. 7). On the other hand, the rates of noradrenaline and adrenaline release in spontaneously hypertensive rats were lower than those in normotensive rats (Tuomisto et al. 1983).

Table 2. Systolic blood pressure in normotensive (Wistar Kyoto) and spontaneously hypertensive rats

	N	Age (Days)	Weight (g)	Systolic Blood Pressure (mm Hg)
WKY	8	60 ± 3	103 ± 11	95 ± 6
SHR	9	60 ± 3	121 ± 4	124 ± 7*

WKY Wistar Kyoto, SHR spontaneous hypertensive rats, N number of experiments. Mean values ± S.E.M. (Tuomisto et al. 1983)

In spontaneously and genetically hypertensive rats, the dopamine level of the hypothalamus was found to be reduced, while the levels of noradrenaline (Fuxe et al. 1979, 1982) and adrenaline (Gianutsos and Moore 1978; Wijnen et al. 1978; Fuxe et al. 1979, 1982) were increased. The catecholamine turnover was not changed (Fuxe et al. 1979, 1982). These findings may also suggest that in the hypothalamus of hypertensive rats, the rate of dopamine release is increased, while the rates of noradrenaline and adrenaline release are decreased. However, care should be taken in interpreting these findings, because many of these determinations were carried out in the whole hypothalamus.

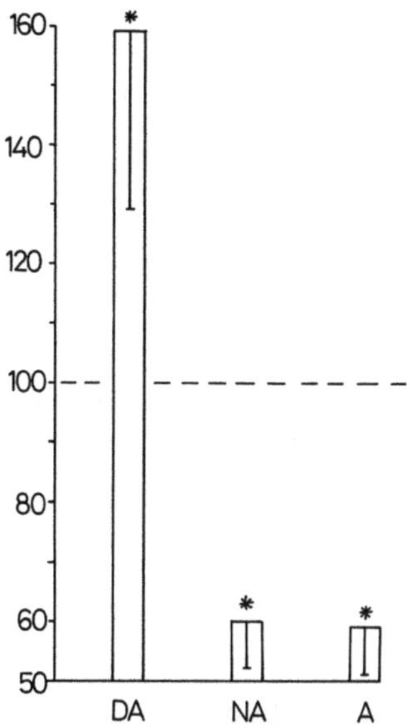

Fig. 7. Resting release of catecholamines in the posterior hypothalamic nucleus of spontaneously hypertensive rats. The release in normotensive (Wistar Kyoto) rat was taken as 100%. *DA* dopamine, *NA* noradrenaline, *A* adrenaline. Mean values of 7–9 experiments ± S.E.M. For differences between normotensive and spontaneously hypertensive rats $^*P < 0.05$. Modified from Tuomisto et al. (1983)

As mentioned above, in anaesthetized cats and in conscious, freely moving rabbits a rise in blood pressure leads to increased release of all three catecholamines in the posterior hypothalamus. Hence, in this hypothalamic region, the released catecholamines seem to possess a hypertensive function. It is plausible that the reduced rates of noradrenaline and adrenaline release in spontaneously hypertensive rats are the consequence of the hypertension, while the enhanced release of dopamine may be the cause or one of the causes for the development of high blood pressure.

Superfusion of the rat hypothalamus with potassium chloride (6×10^{-2} mol/liter) enhanced the rates of release of all three catecholamines (Fig. 8). Potassium chloride increased the release of catecholamines to approximately the same extent in normotensive and hypertensive animals. Thus, the alterations in the rates of release observed in the hypertensive animals (Fig. 7) seem to reflect changes in the neuronal activities rather than changes in the responsiveness of the hypothalamic nerve terminals to stimuli (Tuomisto et al. 1983).

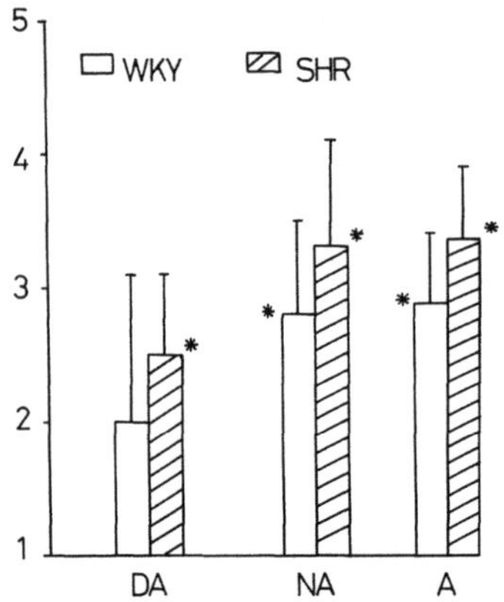

Fig. 8. Release of catecholamines by KCl-rich CSF. *DA* dopamine, *NA* noradrenaline, *A* adrenaline. The superfusate was continuously collected in 10 min periods, the hypothalamus was superfused with KCl-rich (6×10^{-2} mol/liter) CSF for 10 min. The rates of release in the samples before superfusing with KCl-rich CSF were taken as 1. For differences between control samples and samples during superfusion with KCl-rich CSF $*P < 0.05$. Modified from Tuomisto et al. (1983)

References

Coorea FMA, Magro IAS, Peres-Polon VL (1982) CNS mediation of cardiovascular responses to the intracerebroventricular administration of catecholamines. Trend Pharmacol Sci 3: 330-332

Dietl H, Sinha JN, Philippu A (1981a) Presynaptic regulation of the release of catecholamines in the cat hypothalamus. Brain Res 208: 213-218

Dietl H, Eisert A, Kraus A, Philippu A (1981b) The release of endogenous catecholamines in the cat hypothalamus is affected by spinal transection and drugs which change the arterial blood pressure. J Auton Pharmacol 1: 279-286

Fuxe K, Ganten D, Jonsson G, Bolme P, Agnati LF, Andersson K, Goldstein M, Hökfelt T (1979) Evidence for a selective reduction of adrenaline turnover in the dorsal midline area of the caudal medulla oblongata of young spontaneous hypertensive rats. Acta Physiol Scand 107: 397-399

Fuxe K, Vincent M, Andersson K, Härfstrand A, Agnati LF, Sassard J, Benfenati F, Hökfelt T (1982) Selective reduction of adrenaline turnover in the dorsal midline area of the caudal medulla oblongata and increase of hypothalamic adrenaline levels in the Lyon strain of genetically hypertensive rats. Eur J Pharmacol 77: 187-191

Gianutsos G, Moore KE (1978) Epinephrine contents of sympathetic ganglia and brain regions of spontaneously hpyertensive rats of different ages. Proc Soc Exp Biol Med 158: 45-49

Iijima T, Philippu A (1980) Failure of isoprenaline and betareceptor blocking drugs to modify depressor response and bradycardia induced by electrical stimulation of the anterior hypothalamus of cats. Naunyn-Schmiedeberg's Arch Pharmacol 312: 27-30

Kawasaki H, Takasaki K (1986) Central alpha-2 adrenoceptormediated hypertensive response to clonidine in conscious, normotensive rats. J Pharmacol Exp Ther 236: 810-818

Lanzinger I, Kobilansky C, Philippu A (1986) Release of catecholamines in the nucleus tractus solitarii under resting conditions and during experimentally induced blood pressure changes. Naunyn-Schmiedeberg's Arch Pharmacol 332 Suppl R58

Levin BE, Goldstein A, Natelson BH (1978) Ultradian rhythm of plasma noradrenaline in rhesus monkeys. Nature 272: 164-166

Majewski H (1983) Modulation of noradrenaline release through activation of presynaptic β-adrenoreceptors. J Auton Pharmacol 3: 47-60

Philippu A, Kittel E (1977) Presence of beta-adrenoceptors in the hypothalamus; their importance

for the pressor response to hypothalamic stimulation. Naunyn-Schmiedeberg's Arch Pharmacol 297: 219-225
Philippu A, Schartner P (1976) Inhibition by locally applied alpha-adrenoreceptor blocking agents of the depressor response to stimulation of the anterior hypothalamus. Naunyn-Schmiedeberg's Arch Pharmacol 295: 1-7
Philippu A, Stroehl U (1978) Beta-adrenoreceptors of the posterior hypothalamus. Clin Exp Hypertension 1: 25-38
Philippu A, Roensberg W, Przuntek H (1973) Effects of adrenergic drugs on pressor responses to hypothalamic stimulation. Naunyn-Schmiedeberg's Arch Pharmacol 578: 373-386
Philippu A, Demmeler R, Roensberg G (1974) Effects of centrally applied drugs on pressor responses to hypothalamic stimulation. Naunyn-Schmiedeberg's Arch Pharmacol 282: 389-400
Philippu A, Dietl H, Sinha JN (1979) In vivo release of endogenous catecholamines in the hypothalamus. Naunyn-Schmiedebergs Arch Pharmacol 308: 137-142
Philippu A, Dietl H, Sinha JN (1980) Rise in blood pressure increases the release of endogenous catecholamines in the anterior hypothalamus of the cat. Naunyn-Schmiedebergs Arch Pharmacol 310: 237-240
Philippu A, Dietl H, Eisert A (1981) Hypotension alters the release of catecholamines in the hypothalamus of the conscious rabbit. Eur J Pharmacol 69: 519-523
Robinson R, Dietl H, Bald M, Kraus A, Philippu A (1983) Effects of short-lasting and long-lasting blood pressure changes on the release of endogenous catecholamines in the hypothalamus of the conscious, freely moving rabbit. Naunyn-Schmiedebergs Arch Pharmacol 322: 203-209
Sinha JN, Dietl H, Philippu A (1980) Effect of a fall of blood pressure on the release of catecholamines in the hypothalamus. Life Sci 26: 1751-1760
Trolin G (1975) Effects of pentobarbitone and decerebration on the clonidine-induced circulatory changes. Eur J Pharmacol 34: 1-7
Tuomisto L, Yamatodani A, Dietl H, Waldmann U, Philippu A (1983) In vivo release of endogenous catecholamines, histamine and GABA in the hypothalamus of Wistar Kyoto and spontaneously hypertensive rats. Naunyn-Schmiedebergs Arch Pharmacol 323: 183-187
Ueda H, Goshima Y, Misu Y (1983) Presynaptic mediation by α_2-, β_1- and β_2-adrenoceptors of endogenous noradrenaline and dopamine release from slices of rat hypothalamus. Life Sci 33: 371-376
Ueda H, Goshima Y, Kubo T, Misu Y (1984) Adrenaline involvement in the presynamptic β-adrenoceptor-mediated mechanism of dopamine release from slices of the rat hypothalamus. Life Sci 34: 1087-1093
Vlahakos D, Gavras I, Gavras H (1985) Alpha-adrenoceptor agonists applied in the area of the nucleus tractus solitarii in the rat: effect of anaesthesia on cardiovascular responses. Brain Res 347: 372-375
Wijnen HJLM, Palkovits M, De Jong W, Versteeg DHG (1978) Elevated adrenaline content in nuclei of the medulla oblongata and the hypothalamus during the development of spontaneous hypertension. Brain Res 157: 191-195

On the Mechanism and Scope of Adrenoceptor-Mediated Control of Sympathetic Neuro-Effector Transmission: A Model Study

L. Stjärne

Department of Physiology, Karolinska Institutet, 10401 Stockholm, Sweden

Introduction

Initially in this paper a presentation is given of what is currently known about the fashion in which the average individual varicosity of sympathetic neurones (Fig. 1) responds to a suprathreshold electrical stimulus applied to the parent axon. This presentation is followed by a discussion of the scope and mechanisms of local α-adrenoceptor mediated control of the secretory response of the varicosity. The aim of the paper is not to provide a comprehensive review, but to discuss certain key aspects (Cunnane 1984; Stjärne 1981, 1985; Stjärne and Åstrand 1976; for an interesting alternative view of sites and mechanisms for local control of stimulus-secretion coupling in sympathetic nerves, see Bevan et al. 1984).

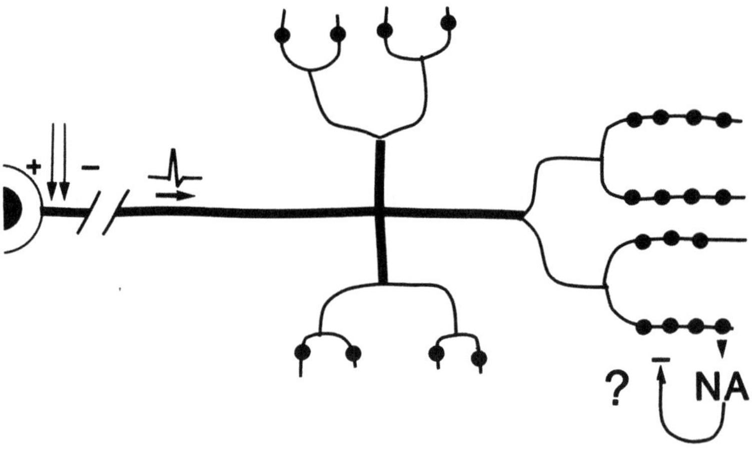

Fig. 1. Idealized sympathetic neurone in rodent vas deferens. Total length of terminals is about 10 cm, with about 20000 potentially secretory varicosities, each containing 500 small and 25 large dense cored vesicles. *NA*, Noradrenaline (Dahlström and Häggendal 1966; Hökfelt 1969; Thuresson-Klein 1983)

New Aspects of the Role of Adrenoceptors in the
Cardiovascular System/Ed. by Grobecker et al.

Secretory Activity of Individual Varicosities

Historical Background: Evidence by Overflow Analysis

The characteristics of the secretory activity of single varicosities have remained unknown owing to a lack of methods which are able to resolve the small amount of transmitter secreted by such tiny structures against the supposedly high background noise from neighbouring varicosities. Folkow et al. (1967) who were the first to formulate an hypothesis based it on studies of the overflow of noradrenaline (NA) evoked by electrical stimulation of sympathetic vasoconstrictor nerves of cat skeletal muscle. When applied to the idealized neurone in Fig. 1, their argument would be the following: The average varicosity contains some 500 vesicles; the amount of transmitter stored in a single vesicle is generally thought to represent the "quantum" (Del Castillo and Katz 1954). If all varicosities are activated by each impulse and secrete one quantum of NA, then (disregarding the possible contribution from the few large dense-cored vesicles) every varicosity and hence the entire population of neurones in the tissue would release 0.2% (1/500) of their NA content. Folkow et al. (1967) found in their experiments that the output per stimulus was about two orders of magnitude lower, or 0.002% of the NA store. This led them to a difficult choice between two mutually exclusive alternatives: (1) If the average varicosity is activated by every stimulus ($P=1$) then the quantum must be small, 1% or less or the contents of a vesicle ($q \leq 0.01$), which would contradict the vesicle hypothesis for quantal secretion; or (2) if the quantum equals the NA contents of a vesicle ($q=1$), then each stimulus would activate only 1% of the varicosities ($P=0.01$). Folkow et al. (1967) preferred the first alternative; Bevan et al. (1969) were the first to argue in favour of the second alternative. Based on studies of NA overflow from the sympathetic nerves of rabbit pulmonary artery, induced by electrical nerve stimulation in the presence of the α-adrenoceptor blocking agent phenoxybenzamine, these authors concluded that the individual varicosity is only intermittently activated, by one out of every 7–8 stimuli, and then secretes a quantum equal to the NA contents of a vesicle ($q=1$; $P=0.13$). Since they used phenoxybenzamine, which enhances NA overflow by about ten-fold in the system used, in controls they would presumably have found the high degree of intermittency predicted in alternative 2 discussed above ($P=0.01$). To make a confident choice between the two alternatives, methods are required which directly resolve the quantum size and/or the probability of activation of individual varicosities. Interesting evidence in support of alternative 2 has been reported by Hirst and Neild (1980). Using a combination of electrophysiological and morphological methods, they found that each electrical stimulus to the sympathetic vasoconstrictor nerves of guinea-pig mesentric arterioles activated only a small fraction, about 1%, of the varicosities. Recently, a novel electrophysiological method has been developed which may resolve directly both P and q in the sympathetic nerves of guinea-pig or mouse vas deferens, on an impulse-by-impulse basis (Blakeley and Cunnane 1979, see below).

New Evidence by Electrophysiological Analysis: "Discrete Events"

Neither overflow or mechanical methods (Fig. 2), nor conventional use of intracellularly recorded excitatory junction potentials (EJPs) resolves the secretory activity of individual release sites of sympathetic nerves. However, analysis of the fluctuations in the rates of rise in EJPs may do so (Blakeley and Cunnane 1979). Under experimental conditions giving optimal resolution (Cunnane and Stjärne 1982, 1984) study of the peaks ["discrete events", (DEs)] in the electronically derived first time differential of the rising phases of fast EJPs (Stjärne and Åstrand 1984) seems to make it possible to directly measure the probability that a nerve impulse will activate the individual release site, and to show it to be in the low range predicted by alternative 2 above ($P = 0.002-0.03$).

The method may also directly resolve q. For most amplitude classes of stimulus-evoked DEs, it is often possible, by visual or computerized image analysis (fingerprinting: see Fig. 3), to find a matching spontaneous DE in the same cell (Cunnane and Stjärne 1982, 1984). Their nearly identical amplitude and time course suggest that both the spontaneous and the evoked DE were caused by the same amount of transmitter (according to the vesicle hypothesis, a single quantum equal to the transmitter contents of a vesicle), secreted from the same or a closely similar site. Repeated appearances of evoked DEs with the same latency amplitude and time course (identical fingerprint) during a stimulus train therefore indicate repeated activation of a particular release site, the characteristic shape of the DE being determined by the distance between the release site and the recording micro-electrode and the impedance of interposed electrically coupled cells.

Figure 3 is a practical example which illustrates that even in cells with complex DE patterns it may be possible to analyse the secretory activity of recognized individual release sites on an impulse-by-impulse basis by studying the occurrence of DEs with identical fingerprints. In this cell, 52 DEs occurred during a train of 100 stimuli. Most of the DEs differed from each other in amplitude and time course. According to the criteria applied in computer image analysis, the 52 DEs belonged

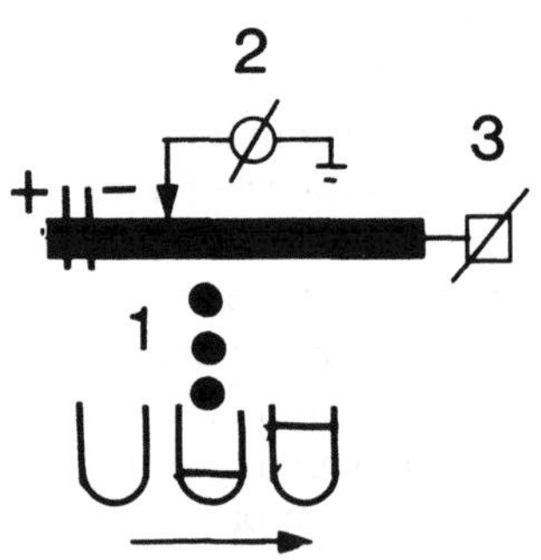

Fig. 2. Methods used to study, directly and indirectly, the secretory response of the individual varicosity of the idealized sympathetic neurone, induced by electrical stimulation. *1*, Overflow of [^{3}H]NA; *2*, intracellular recording in smooth muscle cells: excitatory junction potentials (EJPs), and discrete events (DEs), the first time derivative of the rising phases of EJPs; *3*, contractile response to nerve stimulation

to 38 different classes, 28 of which had only one member while 12 had two members. Shown are, for clarity, only three classes of the paired DEs. Each class is presumed to represent the total stimulus-induced secretory activity of a particular release site. In each class, the probability of activation was 0.02. Many of the non-paired DEs may represent release sites with a probability of 0.01. It cannot be excluded that some of them were caused by fusion of the effects of simultaneous secretion of two or more quanta (the data do not indicate whether in that case they were secreted from the same or from two or more neighbouring varicosities).

There are two main problems connected with the use of DEs to analyse quantal NA secretion: (1) Apparently DEs are not caused by NA, since they may be normal in appearance in NA-depleted preparations. They are abolished by desensitization of ATP receptors (Stjärne and Åstrand 1984) and hence DEs may be caused by ATP co-secreted along with NA, possibly from the same vesicle of sympathetic nerves (Sneddon and Westfall 1984; Sneddon et al. 1982; Meldrum and Burnstock 1983; Stjärne and Åstrand 1984, 1985). In that case DEs caused by the small ATP component of "sympathetic neurotransmitter quanta" (approximately 20 molecules ATP and 1000 molecules NA?; Fredholm et al. 1982) may indirectly also reflect the NA component. (2) The small ATP component of the quantum may be effective (i.e., give rise to DEs) only when it is secreted from varicosities forming close junctions with the impaled smooth muscle cell or its electrically coupled immediate neighbours (Stjärne and Åstrand 1984).

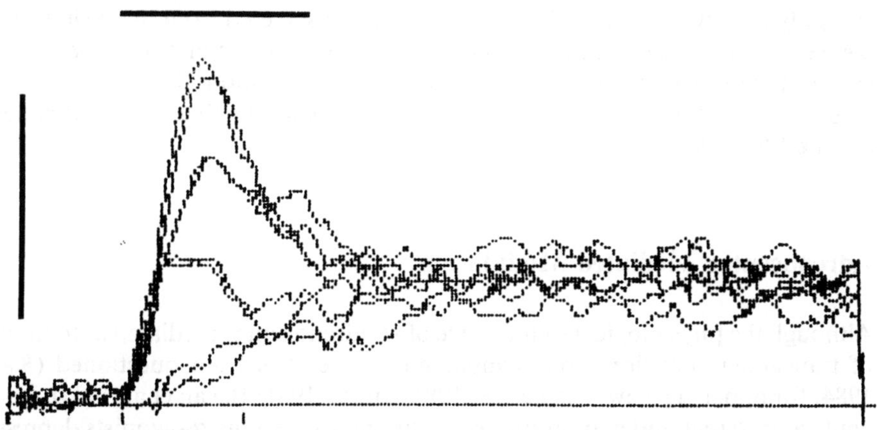

Fig. 3. Three complementary pairs of DEs and two low-amplitude sweeps to indicate background noise. Vertical bar, 1 V/s; *horizontal bar,* 10 ms. In this cell of mouse vas deferens, a train of 100 stimuli (10 V, 0.08 ms; 0.5 Hz; 1.3 m*M* calcium in medium) evoked a total of 52 DEs within the same latency band. Analogue signals on magnetic tape were digitized; data stored on a floppy disc could be recalled from random access memory and displayed on the high-resolution graphics of an ABC 800 microcomputer. A program was developed for computerized recognition of identity of curves. According to the criteria used, within the window indicated by the *bars* at the bottom of the graph, 12 classes of DEs with identical fingerprints were recognized, with two members in each class. For clarity, only three of these classes are shown: class 1 (responses to stimuli 2 and 22 in the train), class 2 (responses to stimuli 13 and 21) and class 3 (responses to stimuli 19 and 81). Each class is believed to reflect the total secretory activity of a particular release site during the train of 100 stimuli

In summary on this point: DEs may be used to monitor quantal NA secretion under two conditions: that ATP and NA are co-secreted in fixed proportions and that the secretory activity of varicosities forming close junctions is representative of that of the average varicosity. In the guinea-pig vas deferens a good correlation has been observed between the overall occurrence of discrete events and the fractional secretion of ^{3}H-NA evoked by comparable stimulation; for those sympathetic nerves these conditions may be fulfilled (Cunnane and Stjärne 1984).

Conclusions Concerning the Secretory Activity of Single Sites

The combined DE and overflow evidence strongly suggests that alternative 2 discussed above is correct. The probability that the secretory mechanisms of the average individual varicosity of the sympathetic nerves of the guinea-pig or mouse vas deferens will be activated by a nerve impulse in the parent axon is low ($P = 0.01$) and whenever activated, the varicosity secretes a single quantum ($q = 1$). In the idealized neurone shown in Fig. 1, under control conditions a nerve stimulus would activate only 200 of its 20000 varicosities; the rest would be silent.

The cause of the extreme intermittency is not fully understood. In part it may be a result of very frequent failure of the nerve impulse to invade the varicosity. However, the intermittency is also due at least in part to restrictive mechanisms in the varicosity itself. Apparently, nerve impulses do not induce secretion from randomly located vesicles; quanta may be immediately available for secretion only when contained in vesicles positioned at preferred release sites, with a capacity for only a few (possibly only two) vesicles. Quanta appear to be secreted from these sites in complementary pairs (see Fig. 3). Secretion of the first quantum of a pair does not autoinhibit that release site, but induces short-lasting facilitation. Release of the second quantum is followed by prolonged secretory silence in that site (Cunnane and Stjärne 1982, 1984).

Adrenoceptor Mediated Modulation

Although the physiological significance of α-adrenoceptor mediated autoinhibition of transmitter secretion from sympathetic nerves has been questioned (Kalsner 1984; for opposing views see Langer 1981; Starke 1981; Bevan et al. 1984), it is generally agreed that under appropriate conditions, exogenous α_2-agonists depress and α_2-antagonists enhance NA secretion from sympathetic nerves in all tissues and species examined.

Scope of α-Autoinhibition

As shown in Fig. 4, typically under control conditions, fractional NA secretion evoked by a nerve impulse is about 0.002% of the tissue content (with some variation). As pointed out by Kalsner and Chan (1979), the fact that this is the level of the

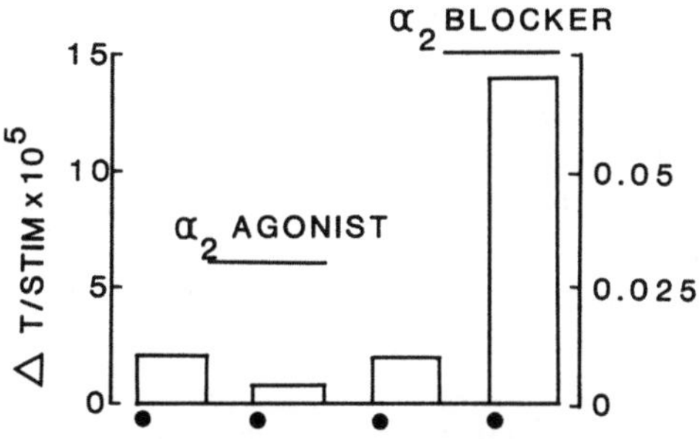

Fig. 4. Typical (in this case fictive) secretory response of the sympathetic nerves of guinea pig or mouse vas deferens to electrical field stimulation at low frequency (1 Hz). Effects of α_2-agonist (e.g., NA at 0.5–1 μ*M*) or α-antagonist (e.g., yohimbine at 1 μ*M*). *Left ordinate*, fractional secretion of [^{3}H]NA per shock. *Right ordinate*, calculated probability that a nerve stimulus to the parent axon would activate the average individual varicosity of the model neurone in Fig. 1, causing it to secrete one quantum of NA. ●, Electrical nerve stimulation

NA output in all tissues, regardless of the width of the neuro-effector clefts is contrary to what would be expected if it is the *intrajunctional* concentration of NA which exerts a feed-back control on the secretory mechanisms, as was earlier believed (Bevan 1977). Also against intrajunctional feedback control speaks the finding in rodent vas deferens that activation of a release site did not locally autoinhibit that site on an impulse-by-impulse basis, but in fact induced short-lasting facilitation, i.e. increased the probability that one of the next few nerve impulses would release the second quantum of a complementary pair (Cunnane and Stjärne 1982, 1984). Therefore it may be the *extrajunctional,* steady-state concentration of NA which autocontrols the secretory mechanisms, by activation of extrajunctional neuronal adrenoceptors (Stjärne 1978; Schipper 1979; Illés and Starke 1983). However, it is still puzzling that the enhancing effect of α-adrenoceptor antagonists is very variable in different tissues and, indeed, seems to be related to the density of innervation and/or the width of junctional clefts (see, for example, Bevan 1977). The problem has not been solved as yet and must therefore be left to additional analysis.

Figure 4 also depicts the typical depressing effect of exogenous α_2-agonist and the enhancing effect of α_2-antagonist on the secretory response to electrical nerve stimulation in tissues such as guinea-pig or mouse vas deferens. As indicated on the right ordinate even when the overall secretory response was increased by about five-fold after blockade of α-autoinhibition (in this example), the secretory response of the average individual varicosity remained intermittent; apparently it still secreted a quantum in response to less than one out of every ten stimuli ($P < 0.1$). The striking secretory intermittency of the individual varicosities under control conditions is thus mainly due other causes than inhibition by autoactivation of presynaptic α-adrenoceptors. Much of the controversy concerning the physiological significance of α-autoinhibition (Kalsner 1984) may be due to failure to appreciate its limited scope, i.e. that it is a system for marginal control. Its purpose may be to locally fine-tune the recruitment of monoquantal units, i.e., to control the probability of activation of individual varicosities only within the range 0.002–0.1 (Stjärne 1985; Stjärne and Åstrand 1986).

Mechanisms of α-Autoinhibition

The sites and mechanisms by which activation of presynaptic α-adrenoceptors depresses transmitter secretion are incompletely understood. The most common assumption is that the receptors are located on the varicosity membrane inside the junctional cleft and that they mediate direct depression of the coupling step in invaded varicosities (depolarization-secretion coupling; see for example Langer 1981; Starke 1981; Bevan et al. 1984). As an alternative, it has been proposed that the receptors occur also extrajunctionally, mediating restriction of the invasion of varicosities (Stjärne 1978; Alberts et al. 1981). In either case, it is assumed that the effect is to a large extent exerted by control of voltage dependent ionic channels in the neuronal membrane, leading to restriction of calcium influx (Horn and MacAfee 1980) or to promotion of potassium efflux (North and Yoshimura 1984). However, evidence has been reported that α-adrenoceptor agonists and antagonists may also act on intraneuronal targets, via second messengers (for a discussion, see Schoffelmeer 1983).

In order to find out whether it is the invasion of varicosities or depolarization-secretion coupling in invaded varicosities which is the immediate target of α-agonists and α-antagonists, their effects on the secretory response to electrical nerve stimulation have been compared with those on the response to stimulation evoked by high concentrations of potassium. The response to electrical nerve stimulation is suppressed by 0.3 μ*M* tetrodotoxin and is therefore not due to direct depolarization of varicosities, but requires sodium channel dependent propagation of nerve impulses, at least in preterminals. In contrast, potassium-evoked secretion is tetrodotoxin resistant and is thus the result of direct depolarization of varicosities. An agent or procedure equally altering the secretory response to both stimuli may be assumed to act mainly on the coupling step; if the effects are more pronounced on electrically evoked secretion, they may be exerted primarily on the invasion of nerve terminals (Stjärne 1978; Alberts et al. 1981).

As shown in Fig. 5, the steady-state secretory responses of the sympathetic nerves in the guinea pig vas deferens to continuous electrical stimulation at 1 Hz and to total depolarization of varicosities with 160 m*M* potassium were relatively similar. Hence, although depolarization is necessary, it is not a sufficient condition for maximal activation of transmitter secretion. Apparently, powerful restrictive mechanisms still prevent uncontrolled release of valuable transmitter even when the varicosity membrane is totally depolarized, although they do not shut off secretion totally. The nature of such control will not be discussed further here.

In Fig. 5 it is also evident that exogenous NA depressed and phentolamine enhanced the secretory responses to electrical stimulation much more than they influenced responses to potassium stimulation. This suggests that the main effect of activation of presynaptic α-adrenoceptors may be to depress the invasion of terminals (Stjärne 1978; Alberts et al. 1981). However, since potassium-induced secretion was also modulated, part of the effect clearly was exerted directly on the varicosities. The remarkable finding that α-agonists and α-antagonists modulated even the secretory response evoked by complete depolarization of varicosities shows that the direct effects on varicosities are exerted on mechanisms other than control of voltage-dependent ionic channels of the varicosity membrane (cf. Schoffelmeer 1983).

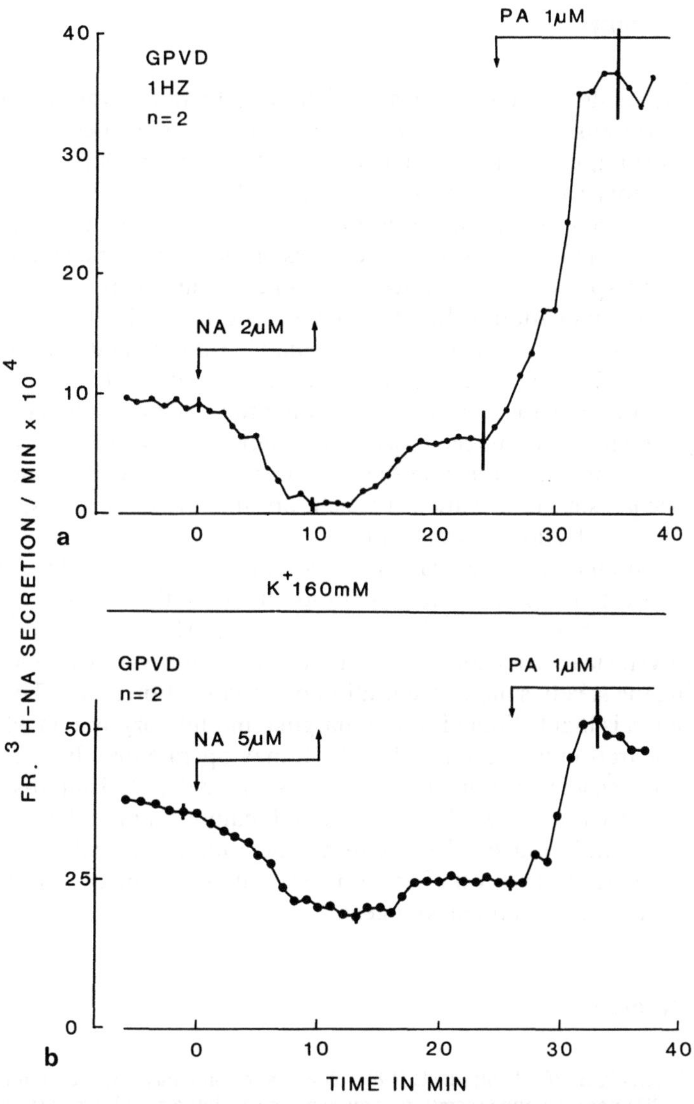

Fig. 5 a, b. Secretory responses of the sympathetic nerves of guinea pig vas deferens *(GPVD)* **a** to continuous electrical field stimulation at 1 Hz or **b** to addition of potassium 160 m*M* to depolarize totally all varicosities (in control experiments by addition of sucrose it was shown that the hypertonicity in itself did not significantly change either the resting efflux or the electrically evoked secretion of labelled transmitter). Effects of exogenous NA and of phentolamine *(PA)* are demonstrated. At time 0 the stimulation had been applied for 10 min. For details concerning the method employed, see Alberts et al. (1981). Desmethylimipramine 0.6 μ*M* and normetanephrine 10 μ*M* were present in the medium to block reuptake of liberated NA. The response to electrical stimulation was totally suppressed by 0.3 μ*M* tetrodotoxin, while potassium-induced secretion was tetrodotoxin resistant; both were abolished when calcium was removed from the medium

Summary

The results seem to support the following tentative working model for sympathetic neurotransmission at the level of individual varicosities and junctions: Basically, a nerve impulse in the axon activates only a very small proportion of the potentially secretory varicosities (P in the range of 0.002–0.03). Whenever activated, the varicosity secretes one quantum only, corresponding to the transmitter contents of a vesicle. Hence, the 20000 varicosities of the neurone behave as a digital, binary system; response of each varicosity to a nerve impulse is either 1 or 0 ("one-or-none"), Upon stimulation at low frequency, long intervals (up to minutes) may pass between successive releases of single quanta (or pairs) into one and the same junctional cleft. Hence, the effect of repetitive stimulation is not to cause accumulation of transmitter in the same cleft, but rather to recruit other junctions also operating in a digital manner. The secretory intermittency may be due in part to frequent failure of nerve impulses to invade the varicosity, but in part it is due to built-in restrictive mechanisms in the varicosity itself, presumably serving as safety devices to prevent uncontrolled loss of transmitter.

Modulation of transmitter secretion is also digital and consists in ± recruitment of one-or-none units. Autoinhibition by activation of presynaptic α-adrenoceptors is only a minor cause of the secretory intermittency. This control mechanism is not driven via intrajunctional receptors, but possibly via extrajunctional receptors, sensing the steady-state concentration of extrajunctional NA. The scope of α-autoinhibition is highly limited; it is a marginal modulatory system which may help to fine-tune transmitter secretion locally. It may operate mainly by restricting the invasion of varicosities, but in part also depresses the depolarization-secretion coupling step in varicosities. The effects are exerted mainly via modulation of voltage-dependent ionic conductances of the neuronal membrane, particularly to calcium and potassium. Part of the direct effects on varicosities may be by another mechanism, via intraneuronal second messengers.

References

Alberts P, Bartfai T, Stjärne L (1981) Site(s) and ionic basis of α-autoinhibition and facilitation of (^{3}H)-noradrenaline secretion in guinea-pig vas deferens. J Physiol (Lond) 312: 297–334

Bevan JA (1977) Some functional consequences of variation in adrenergic synaptic cleft width and in nerve density and distribution. Fed Proc 36: 2439–2443

Bevan JA, Chesher GB, Su C (1969) Release of adrenergic transmitter from terminal nerve plexus in artery. Agents Actions 1: 20–26

Bevan JA, Tayo FM, Rowan RA, Bevan RD (1984) Presynaptic α-receptor control of adrenergic transmitter release in blood vessels. Fed Proc 43: 1365–1370

Blakeley AGH, Cunnane TC (1979) The packeted release of transmitter from the sympathetic nerves of the guinea-pig vas deferens: an electrophysiological study. J Physiol (Lond) 296: 85–96

Cunnane TC (1984) The mechanism of neurotransmitter release from sympathetic nerves. TINS 7: 248–253

Cunnane TC, Stjärne L (1982) Secretion of transmitter from individual varicosities of guinea-pig and mouse vas deferens: all-or-none and extremely intermittent. Neuroscience 7: 2565–2576

Cunnane TC, Stjärne L (1984) Transmitter secretion from individual varicosities of guinea-pig and mouse vas deferens: highly intermittent and monoquantal. Neuroscience 13: 1–20

Dahlström A, Häggendal J (1966) Some quantitative studies on the noradrenaline content in the cell bodies and terminals of a sympathetic adrenergic neuron system. Acta Physiol Scand 67: 271-277

Del Castillo J, Katz B (1954) Quantal components of the end-plate potential. J Physiol (Lond) 124: 560-573

Folkow B, Häggendal J, Lisander B (1967) Extent of release and elimination of noradrenaline at peripheral adrenergic nerve terminals. Acta Physiol Scand [Suppl] 307: 1-38

Fredholm BB, Fried G, Hedqvist P (1982) Origin of adenosine released from rat vas deferens by nerve stimulation. Eur J Pharmacol 79: 233-243

Hirst GDS, Neild TO (1980) Some properties of spontaneous excitatory junction potentials recorded from arterioles of guinea-pig. J Physiol (Lond) 303: 43-60

Horn JP, MacAfee DA (1980) Alpha-adrenergic inhibition of calcium-dependent potentials in rat sympathetic neurones. J Physiol (Lond) 301: 191-204

Hökfelt T (1969) Distribution of noradrenaline storing particles in peripheral adrenergic neurons as revealed by electron microscopy. Acta Physiol Scand 76: 427-440

Illés P, Starke K (1983) An electrophysiological study of presynaptic α-adrenoceptors in the vas deferens of the mouse. Br J Pharmacol 78: 365-373

Kalsner S (1984) Symposium on "The noradrenergic presynaptic receptor controversy". Fed Proc 43: 1351-1381

Kalsner S, Chan CC (1979) Adrenergic antagonists and the presynaptic receptor hypothesis in vascular tissue. J Pharmacol Exp Ther 211: 257-264

Langer SZ (1981) Presynaptic regulation of the release of catecholamines. Pharmacol Rev 32: 337-362

Meldrum LA, Burnstock G (1983) Evidence that ATP acts as a cotransmitter with noradrenaline in the sympathetic nerves supplying the guinea-pig vas deferens. Eur J Pharmacol 92: 161-163

North RA, Yoshimura M (1984) The actions of noradrenaline on neurones of the rat substantia gelatinosa in vitro. J Physiol (Lond) 349: 43-55

Schipper J (1979) A scanning microfluorimetric study on noradrenergic neurotransmission. Thesis Rodopi, Amsterdam

Schoffelmeer T (1983) Presynaptic alpha-adrenoceptors and neurotransmitter release from central noradrenergic neurons. Thesis, Rodopi, Amsterdam

Sneddon P, Westfall DP (1984) Pharmacological evidence that adenosine triphosphate and noradrenaline are co-transmitters in the guinea-pig vas deferens. J Physiol (Lond) 347: 561-580

Sneddon P, Westfall DP, Fedan JS (1982) Cotransmitters in the motor nerves of the guinea-pig vas deferens: electrophysiological evidence. Science (NY) Am 218: 693-695

Starke K (1981) Presynaptic receptors. Ann Rev Pharmacol Toxicol 21: 7-30

Stjärne L (1978) Facilitation and receptor-mediated regulation of noradrenaline secretion by control of recruitment of varicosities as well as by control of electro-secretory coupling. Neuroscience 3: 1147-1155

Stjärne L (1981) On sites and mechanisms of presynaptic control of noradrenaline secretion. In: Stjärne L, Hedqvist P, Lagercrantz H, Wennmalm Å (eds) Chemical neurotransmission 75 years. Academic Press, London, pp 257-272

Stjärne L (1985) Scope and mechanisms of control of stimulus-secretion coupling in single varicosities of sympathetic nerves. Clin Sci 68 [Suppl 10]: 77s-81s

Stjärne L, Åstrand P (1984) Discrete events measure single quanta of ATP secreted from sympathetic nerves of guinea-pig and mouse vas deferens. Neuroscience 13: 21-28

Stjärne L, Åstrand P (1985) Relative pre- and postjunctional roles of noradrenaline and adenosine 5′-triphosphate as neurotransmitters of the sympathetic nerves of guinea-pig and mouse vas deferens. Neuroscience 14: 929-946

Stjärne L, Åstrand P (1985a) Sites of action of presynaptic inhibition mediated via adrenoceptors. In: Proceedings from symposium on 'Pharmacology of adrenoceptors', August 1984, University of Manchester. Macmillan, pp 157-166

Thuresson-Klein Å (1983) Exocytosis from large and small dense cored vesicles in noradrenergic nerve terminals. Neuroscience 10: 245-252

Presynaptic α-Adrenoceptor Control of Transmitter Release from Vascular Sympathetic Neurones in Vitro*

O. A. Nedergaard

Department of Pharmacology, Odense University School of Medicine, J. B. Winsløws Vej 19, 5000 Odense C, Denmark

Introduction

The documentation for the observation that depolarization-evoked adrenergic transmitter release from sympathetic neurones is decreased by α_2-adrenoceptor agonists, while it is enhanced by α_2-adrenoceptor antagonists seems overwhelming (Langer 1977, 1981; Starke 1977, 1981; Westfall 1977; Gillespie 1980; Vizi 1979). This has led to the autoreceptor theory, according to which noradrenaline release from sympathetic neurones is modulated by the neurogenic transmitter itself: activation of presynaptic α_2-adrenoceptors initiates a negative feedback system which results in subsequent inhibition of transmitter release. Recently, this hypothesis has been challenged (Chan and Kalsner 1979; Kalsner 1979, 1980a, 1980b, 1981, 1982a, 1982b, 1983; Angus and Korner 1980; Angus et al. 1984).

The present study was undertaken in order to obtain more insight into the physiological relevance of presynaptic α_2-adrenoceptors. This was done by studying the effect of α-adrenoceptor antagonists on the release of noradrenaline evoked by nerve stimulation of rabbit pulmonary artery at several frequencies in the presence of various inhibitors of inactivation pathways.

Methods

The method previously described in detail by (Nedergaard (1980) was used. Briefly, rings of rabbit pulmonary artery were incubated with (–)-^{3}H-noradrenaline (^{3}H-NA). After a wash-out period, the arteries were subjected to electrical-field stimulation (300 pulses, 0.5 ms, 225 mA, 3 Hz, unless otherwise remarked) up to seven times (S_1–S_7). S_3 (=100%) was used as control. The ^{3}H-overflow was collected in fractions (2 ml) every 2 min. In some experiments, cocaine and corticosterone were added to the salt solution to reduce neuronal and extraneuronal uptake respectively.

* Supported by P. Carl Petersen's Fund and the Novo Foundation

New Aspects of the Role of Adrenoceptors in the Cardiovascular System/Ed. by Grobecker et al.

Results

Effect of Inhibitors of Transmitter Uptake and Enzymatic Degradation on Stimulation-Evoked Transmitter Overflow

Pargyline ($3 \times 10^{-4} M$), an inhibitor of monoamine oxidase (MAO), increased the ^{3}H-overflow evoked by field stimulation of rabbit pulmonary artery preloaded with ^{3}H-NA at 1 and 3 Hz and decreased it at 30 Hz (Fig. 1). U-0521 (3′,4′-dihydroxy-2-methylpropiophenone; $3 \times 10^{-6} M$), an inhibitor of catechol-*O*-methyltransferase (COMT), enhanced the overflow at 1 Hz and reduced it at 30 Hz (Fig. 1). Corticosterone ($4 \times 10^{-5} M$) did not alter the stimulation-evoked overflow at any frequency (1–30 Hz) tested (Fig. 2). Cocaine ($3 \times 10^{-6} M$) enhanced the ^{3}H overflow slightly at 1–30 Hz (Fig. 2). At $3 \times 10^{-5} M$, cocaine enhanced the ^{3}H overflow at 1 Hz (48%) and reduced it at 30 Hz (34%; Fig. 2). Corticosterone ($4 \times 10^{-5} M$) did not modify this effect (Fig. 2).

Effect of α-Adrenoceptor Antagonists on Stimulation-Evoked Transmitter Overflow and Modulation thereof by Inhibitors of Uptake Mechanisms and Enzymes

Phenoxybenzamine ($10^{-6} M$) and chlorpromazine ($3 \times 10^{-6} M$) potentiated the stimulation-evoked ^{3}H overflow at 1–30 Hz (Fig. 3). Phenoxybenzamine caused a much

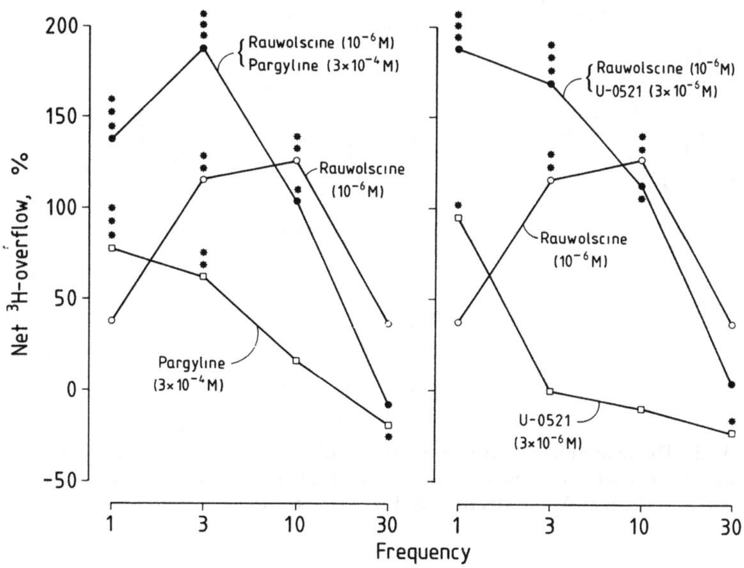

Fig. 1. Modulation by inhibitors of MAO and COMT of the relationship between frequency of stimulation and the effect of rauwolscine on ^{3}H overflow evoked by electrical-field stimulation of rabbit isolated pulmonary artery preloaded with ^{3}H-NA. The data represent mean net ^{3}H overflow (drug-treated-untreated tissue) expressed as a percentage of values derived from untreated tissues. The level of significant differences between drug-treated and control groups are: *, $P < 0.05$; **, $P < 0.01$; ***, $P < 0.001$ ($n = 6$–9)

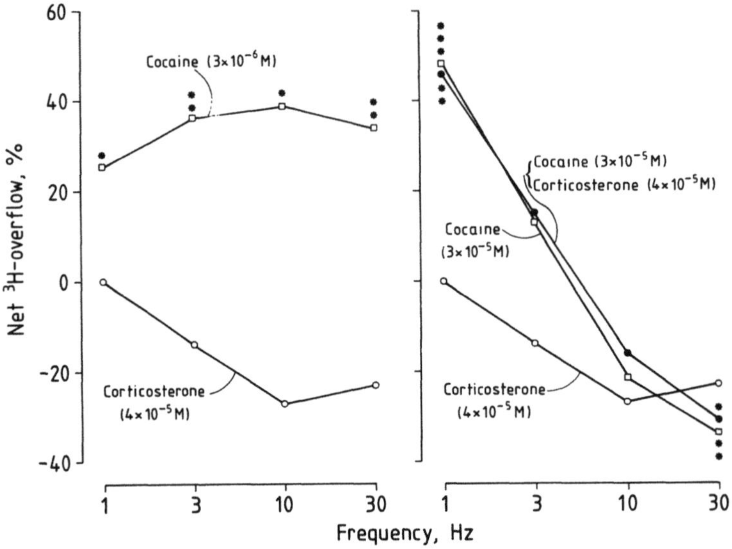

Fig. 2. The relationship between frequency of stimulation and the effect of inhibitors of uptake-1 and -2 on ^{3}H overflow evoked by electrical-field stimulation of rabbit isolated pulmonary artery preloaded with ^{3}H-NA. For details, see Fig. 1

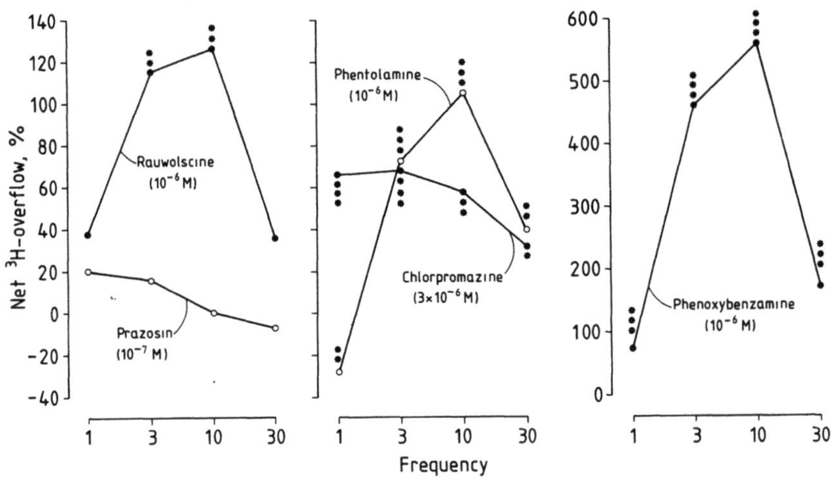

Fig. 3. The relationship between frequency of stimulation and the effect of α-adrenoceptor antagonists on ^{3}H overflow evoked by electrical-field stimulation of rabbit isolated pulmonary artery preloaded with ^{3}H-NA. For details, see Fig. 1 ($n = 6-10$)

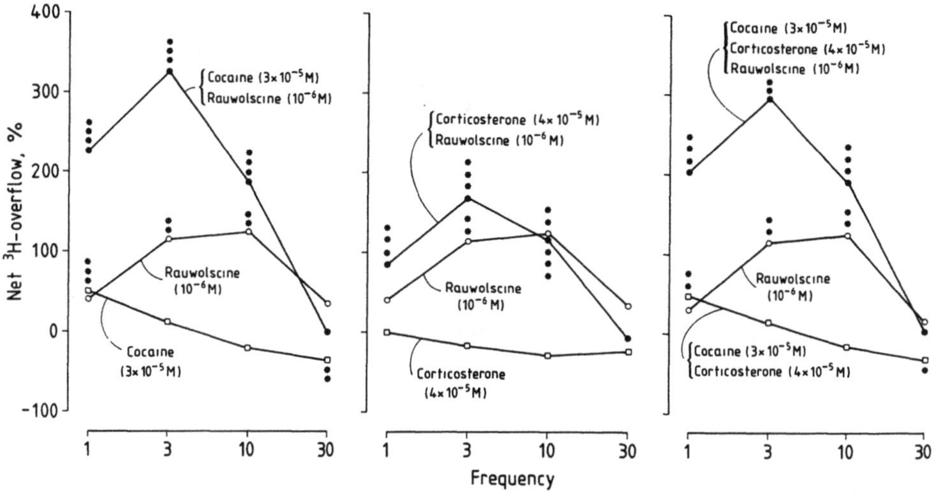

Fig. 4. Modulation by inhibitors of uptake-1 and -2 of the relationship between frequency of stimulation and the effect of rauwolscine on ^{3}H overflow evoked by electrical-field stimulation of rabbit isolated pulmonary artery preloaded with ^{3}H-NA. For details, see Fig. 1 ($n = 6$–7)

higher enhancement than chlorpromazine. The maximum potentiation was seen at 10 Hz (499%) in the case of phenoxybenzamine and at 3 Hz (68%) for chlorpromazine. Phentolamine (10^{-6} *M*) decreased the ^{3}H overflow at 1 Hz and enhanced it at 3–30 Hz (Fig. 3); the maximum enhancement was seen at 10 Hz. Rauwolscine (10^{-6} *M*) enhanced the stimulation-evoked ^{3}H overflow maximally at 10 Hz (126%) and had no effect at 1 and 30 Hz (Fig. 3).

The ability of inhibitors of transmitter uptake systems and of metabolic enzymes to influence the enhancing effect of rauwolscine (10^{-6} *M*) was examined (Figs. 1, 4). Cocaine (3×10^{-5} *M*), cocaine (3×10^{-5} *M*) + corticosterone (4×10^{-5} *M*), pargyline (3×10^{-4} *M*) and U-0521 (3×10^{-6} *M*) increased the rauwolscine-induced enhancement at 1 and 3 Hz, but had no influence at 10 and 30 Hz.

Discussion

Inactivation of noradrenaline released by nerve stimulation in blood vessels is mainly carried out by neuronal and extraneuronal uptake of the transmitter and subsequent inactivation by MAO and COMT (Osswald and Guimarães 1983). The uptake mechanisms for noradrenaline can thus regulate the fraction of transmitter to activate presynaptic α_2-adrenoceptors (Langer 1981).

When cocaine was used in a ten fold lower concentration (3×10^{-6} *M*) than that usually employed in presynaptic receptor studies in order to cause maximal inhibition of neuronal uptake without compromising the release process itself (Schrold and Nedergaard 1979), this uptake inhibitor enhanced the ^{3}H overflow evoked by stimulation of pulmonary artery preloaded with ^{3}H-NA. The enhancement is probably due to the partial removal of an inactivation pathway. As a result, more ^{3}H-NA escapes from the synaptic cleft and is collected in the ^{3}H overflow. According to this proposal, the cleft concentration of ^{3}H-NA is insufficient to activate presynaptic α_2-adrenoceptors. This may well be due to the fact that the synaptic cleft in rabbit pulmonary artery is wide (Bevan 1977). When a ten-fold higher concentration of cocaine ($3 \times 10^{-5} M$) was used, the enhancement was retained at 1 Hz, while the ^{3}H overflow was reduced at 30 Hz. This suggests that as the frequency of stimulation was increased, the intrasynaptic cleft concentration of ^{3}H-NA became concomitantly larger, which resulted in a correspondingly greater activation of presynaptic inhibitory α-adrenoceptors. Consequently, a high degree of neuronal uptake inhibition by cocaine leads to enhanced feedback inhibition when the stimulation frequency is sufficiently high. This view is in line with that expressed by other authors (Cubeddu et al. 1974; Dubocovich and Langer 1976; Langer 1981).

Corticosterone, a highly selective inhibitor of extraneuronal uptake (Iversen and Salt 1970) altered neither the stimulation-evoked ^{3}H overflow nor the effect of cocaine on this process (Fig. 2). This indicates that extraneuronal uptake does not play an important role in determining the intrasynaptic cleft concentration of noradrenaline released by nerve action potentials even when neuronal uptake is inhibited.

In series with neuronal and extraneuronal uptake, MAO and COMT participate in the inactivation of noradrenaline. Pargyline and U-0521 are inhibitors of MAO and of COMT, respectively. Each of these compounds enhanced and decreased the ^{3}H overflow at a low and high frequency, respectively (Fig. 1). The simplest explanation for these findings is the same as offered above for cocaine: at a low frequency (1 Hz), removal of either inactivation pathway results in more unchanged ^{3}H-transmitter in the ^{3}H overflow. As the frequency is increased stepwise to 30 Hz, the negative feedback system is activated more and more, owing to an increase in the perineuronal ^{3}H-NA concentration. The enhancement of ^{3}H overflow seen with U-0521 is surprising, since corticosterone had no effect. It may be surmised, however, that extraneuronal COMT localized in the adventitia of pulmonary artery may be of importance in regulating the perineuronal transmitter concentration. COMT is present and functional in adventitia (Verity et al. 1972; Levin 1974; Schrold and Nedergaard 1981).

The present results confirm that the stimulation-evoked release of ^{3}H-NA from rabbit pulmonary artery is enhanced by rauwolscine (Weitzell et al. 1979), phentolamine (Starke et al. 1974, 1975; Borowski et al. 1977) and phenoxybenzamine (Su and Bevan 1970). The enhancing effect of these α-adrenoceptor antagonists depended on the frequency of stimulation (Fig. 3): the ^{3}H overflow was enhanced concomitantly with an increase in frequency from 1 to 10 Hz. This is consistent with the view that the effectiveness of α-adrenoceptor antagonists in enhancing the release of noradrenaline is dependent on the presence of a sufficient perineuronal concentration of transmitter to activate presynaptic α_2-adrenoceptors (Cubeddu and Weiner 1975; Story et al. 1981; Auch-Schwelk et al. 1983). Rauwolscine had no effect at 1 Hz (Fig. 3). At this low frequency, the presynaptic α_2-adrenoceptors were presumably not activated sufficiently for a measurable disinhibition by rauwolscine. As the frequency was increased stepwise from 1 to 10 Hz, presumably the biophase concentration of ^{3}H-NA became correspondingly higher. As a result, autoinhibition was intensified, and hence, an increasing effect of rauwolscine was observed.

If the failure of rauwolscine to enhance the ^{3}H overflow at 1 Hz is due to an insufficient perineuronal amount of ^{3}H-NA, then the removal of neuronal accumulation should lead to an increase in the biophase concentration of transmitter and, in turn, to an augmentation in the release-enhancing effect of rauwolscine. This was indeed found. Cocaine, a well-known inhibitor of neuronal uptake, augmented the rauwolscine-induced enhancement of ^{3}H overflow at both 1 and 3 Hz. The results obtained with rauwolscine and cocaine, either alone or in combination, are clearly in support of the autoreceptor hypothesis.

Cocaine reduced the peak enhancement of ^{3}H overflow seen with rauwolscine at 10 Hz (Fig. 4). This reduction is probably due to the displacement of rauwolscine from the presynaptic α_2-adrenoceptor by the increased amount of ^{3}H-NA in the biophase, as a result of the removal of the neuronal inactivation pathway. This also would correspond to the autoreceptor hypothesis.

Corticosterone increased rauwolscine-induced enhancement to a much lesser extent (Fig. 4). This was the case even when neuronal uptake was inhibited by cocaine (Fig. 4). This again suggests that extraneuronal accumulation under the present experimental conditions plays a minor role in determining the perineuronal concentration of released transmitter. The wide synaptic cleft in the pulmonary artery (Bevan 1977) is probably a contributing factor.

The positive interaction between rauwolscine and either pargyline or U-0521 (Fig. 1) can be explained in the same manner as for cocaine (vide supra). The ability of U-0521 to modify the effect of rauwolscine is somewhat surprising, since corticosterone had little effect. It may be speculated that U-0521 inhibits a corticosterone-insensitive enzymatic site of loss located extraneuronally in the adventitia. More work is required to settle this point.

The non-selective α-adrenoceptor antagonist phentolamine reduced the ^{3}H overflow at 1 Hz (Fig. 3). This supports the view that phentolamine acts as a partial agonist (Limberger and Starke 1984).

The enhancement of stimulation-evoked ^{3}H overflow seen with chlorpromazine (Fig. 3) is probably due to a cocaine-like effect of this drug. Chlorpromazine is a potent inhibitor of neuronal uptake of noradrenaline (Abrahamsen and Nedergaard 1981).

Phenoxybenzamine, a non-selective α-adrenoceptor antagonist, caused a severalfold higher enhancement of ^{3}H overflow evoked by stimulation (Fig. 3). This is probably due to the fact that phenoxybenzamine is a potent irreversible inhibitor of neuronal and extraneuronal uptake.

The frequency-response curves for rauwolscine, phentolamine and phenoxybenzamine were bell-shaped (Fig. 3). At the high stimulation frequency (30 Hz), rauwolscine did not enhance ^{3}H overflow, while phentolamine and phenoxybenzamine did, but to a much lesser extent than the peak values at 10 Hz. One explanation for these observations may be that the biophase concentration of released transmitter became so large that the antagonists in the concentrations used could no longer protect the presynaptic α_2-adrenoceptors against autoinhibition. This explanation is probably not valid for phenoxybenzamine, since this agent causes irreversible blockade. Another possibility is that at 30 Hz, the autoinhibition system either no longer functions or functions to a lesser degree than at lower frequencies.

Summary

The modulating role of presynaptic α_2-adrenoceptors on transmitter release from vascular sympathetic neurones was examined. This was done by examining how removing inactivation pathways influences the effect of α-adrenoceptor antagonists on the release of transmitter from noradrenergic neurones. Rabbit isolated main pulmonary artery preloaded with ^{3}H-noradrenaline (^{3}H-NA) was used.

Pargyline (3×10^{-4} *M*) increased the stimulation-evoked ^{3}H overflow at 1 and 3 Hz and decreased it at 30 Hz. U-0521 (3′,4′-dihydroxy-2-methyl-propiophenone; 3×10^{-6} *M*) enhanced the overflow at 1 Hz and had no effect at 3–30 Hz. Corticosterone (4×10^{-5} *M*) did not alter the stimulation-evoked overflow at 1–30 Hz. Cocaine (3×10^{-6} *M*) enhanced the ^{3}H overflow slightly at 1–30 Hz. At 3×10^{-5} *M*, cocaine enhanced the ^{3}H overflow at 1 Hz and reduced it at 30 Hz. Corticosterone did not modify this effect.

Phenoxybenzamine (10^{-6} *M*) and chlorpromazine (3×10^{-6} *M*) potentiated the stimulation-evoked ^{3}H overflow at 1–30 Hz. Phentolamine (10^{-6} *M*) decreased the ^{3}H overflow at 1 Hz and enhanced it at 3–30 Hz. Rauwolscine (10^{-6} *M*) enhanced the stimulation-evoked ^{3}H overflow maximally at 10 Hz and had no effect at 1 and 30 Hz.

Cocaine (3×10^{-5} *M*), cocaine (3×10^{-5} *M*) + corticosterone (4×10^{-5} *M*), pargyline (3×10^{-4} *M*) and U-0521 (3×10^{-6} *M*) increased the rauwolscine-induced enhancement at 1 and 3 Hz, but had no influence at 10 and 30 Hz.

The main conclusion is that the biophase concentration of noradrenaline released from sympathetic neurones regulates its own release via presynaptic α_2-adrenoceptors.

References

Abrahamsen J, Nedergaard OA (1981) Effect of chlorpromazine on adrenergic neuroeffector transmission in isolated blood vessels. Br J Pharmacol 74: 943P–944P

Angus J, Korner PI (1980) Evidence against presynaptic α-adrenoceptor modulation of cardiac sympathetic transmission. Nature 286: 288–291

Angus JA, Bobik A, Jackman GP, Kopin IJ, Korner PI (1984) Role of autoinhibitory feed-back in cardiac sympathetic transmission assessed by simultaneous measurements of changes in ^{3}H-efflux and atrial rate in guinea-pig atrium. Br J Pharmacol 81: 201–204

Auch-Schwelk W, Starke K, Steppeler A (1983) Experimental conditions required for the enhancement by α-adrenoceptor antagonists of noradrenaline release in the rabbit ear artery. Br J Pharmacol 78: 543–551

Bevan JA (1977) Some functional consequences of variation in adrenergic synaptic cleft width and in nerve density and distribution. Fed Proc 36: 2439–2443

Borowski E, Starke K, Ehrl H, Endo T (1977) A comparison of pre- and postsynaptic effects of α-adrenolytic drugs in the pulmonary artery of the rabbit. Neuroscience 2: 285–296

Chan CC, Kalsner S (1979) An examination of the negative feedback function of presynaptic adrenoceptors in a vascular tissue. Br J Pharmacol 67: 401–407

Cubeddu XL, Weiner N (1975) Nerve stimulation-mediated overflow of norepinephrine and dopamine-β-hydroxylase. III. Effects of norepinephrine depletion of the α-presynaptic regulation of release. J Pharmacol Exp Ther 192: 1–14

Cubeddu XL, Barnes EM, Langer SZ, Weiner N (1974) Release of norepinephrine and dopamine-β-hydroxylase by nerve stimulation. I. Role of neuronal and extraneuronal uptake and of α-presynaptic receptors. J Pharmacol Exp Ther 190: 431-450

Dubocovich ML, Langer SZ (1976) Influence of the frequency of nerve stimulation on the metabolism of ^{3}H-norepinephrine released from the perfused cat spleen: differences observed during and after the period of stimulation. J Pharmacol Exp Ther 198: 83-101

Gillespie JS (1980) Presynaptic receptors in the autonomic nervous system. In: Szekeres L (ed) Adrenergic activators and inhibitors. Springer, Berlin Heidelberg New York, pp 353-425 Handbook of experimental pharmacology, vol 54/I

Iversen LL, Salt PJ (1970) Inhibition of catecholamine uptake by steroids in the isolated rat heart. Br J Pharmacol 40: 528-530

Kalsner S (1979) Single pulse stimulation of guinea-pig vas deferens and the presynaptic receptor hypothesis. Br J Pharmacol 66: 343-349

Kalsner S (1980a) Limitations of presynaptic adrenoceptor theory: the characteristics of the effect of noradrenaline and phenoxybenzamine on stimulation-induced efflux of [^{3}H]-noradrenaline in vas deferens. J Pharmacol Exp Ther 212: 232-239

Kalsner (1980b) The effect of (+)- and (−)-propranolol on ^{3}H-transmitter efflux in guinea-pig atria and the presynaptic β-adrenoceptor hypothesis. Br J Pharmacol 70: 491-498

Kalsner S (1981) The role of calcium in the effects of noradrenaline and phenoxybenzamine on adrenergic transmitter release from atria: No support for negative feedback of release. Br J Pharmacol 73: 363-371

Kalsner S (1982a) Evidence against the unitary hypotheses of agonist and antagonist action at presynaptic adrenoceptors. Br J Pharmacol 77: 375-380

Kalsner S (1982b) Feedback regulation of neurotransmitter release through adrenergic presynaptic receptors: time for a reassessment. In: Kalsner S (ed) Trends in autonomic pharmacology, vol 2. Urban and Schwarzenberg, Baltimore, pp 385-425

Kalsner S (1983) Yohimbine and prolongation of stimulation pulse duration alter similarly ^{3}H-transmitter efflux in heart: an alternative to the negative feedback hypothesis. Br J Pharmacol 79: 985-992

Langer SZ (1977) Presynaptic receptors and their role in the regulation of transmitter release. Br J Pharmacol 60: 481-497

Langer SZ (1981) Presynaptic regulation of the release of catecholamines. Pharmacol Rev 81: 337-362

Levin J (1974) The uptake and metabolism of ^{3}H-L- and ^{3}H-DL-norepinephrine by intact rabbit aorta and by isolated adventitia and media. J Pharmacol Exp Ther 190: 210-226

Limberger N, Starke K (1984) Further study of prerequisites for the enhancement by α-adrenoceptor antagonists of the release of noradrenaline. Naunyn-Schmiedebergs Arch Pharmacol 325: 240-246

Nedergaard OA (1980) Modulation by the muscarinic agonist McN-A-343 of noradrenaline release from vascular sympathetic neurones. J Cardiovasc Pharmacol 2: 629-643

Osswald W, Guimarães S (1983) Adrenergic mechanisms in blood vessels: morphological and pharmacological aspects. Rev Physiol Biochem Pharmacol 96: 53-122

Schrold J, Nedergaard OA (1979) Frequency-dependence of the metabolism of ^{3}H-noradrenaline release from rabbit isolated aorta: effects of a combination of cocaine and corticosterone or hydrocortisone. Acta Pharmacol Toxicol 44: 13-21

Schrold J, Nedergaard OA (1981) Effect of cocaine and corticosterone on the metabolism of ^{3}H-noradrenaline release from rabbit isolated aorta and adventitia. Acta Pharmacol Toxicol 48: 233-241

Starke K (1977) Regulation of noradrenaline release by presynaptic receptor systems. Rev Physiol Biochem Pharmacol 77: 1-124

Starke K (1981) Presynaptic receptors. Ann Rev Pharmacol Toxicol 21: 7-30

Starke K, Montel H, Gayk W, Merker R (1974) Comparison of the effects of clonidine on pre- and postsynaptic adrenoceptors in the rabbit pulmonary artery. Naunyn-Schmiedebergs Arch Pharmacol 285: 133-150

Starke K, Endo T, Taube HD (1975) Relative pre- and postsynaptic potencies of α-adrenoceptor agonists in the rabbit pulmonary artery. Naunyn-Schmiedebergs Arch Pharmacol 291: 55-78

Story DF, McCulloch MW, Rand MJ, Stanford-Starr CA (1981) Conditions required for the inhibitory feedback loop in noradrenergic transmission. Nature 293: 62-65
Su C, Bevan JA (1970) The release of ^{3}H-norepinephrine in arterial strips studied by the technique of superfusion and transmural stimulation. J Pharmacol Exp Ther 172: 62-68
Verity MA, Su C, Bevan JA (1972) Transmural and subcellular localization of monoamine oxidase and catechol-*O*-methyltransferase in rabbit aorta. Biochem Pharmacol 21: 193-201
Vizi ES (1979) Presynaptic modulation of neurochemical transmission. Progr Neurobiol 12: 181-290
Weitzell R, Tanaka T, Starke K (1979) Pre- and postsynaptic effects of yohimbine stereoisomers on noradrenergic transmission in the pulmonary artery of the rabbit. Naunyn-Schmiedebergs Arch Pharmacol 308: 127-136
Westfall TC (1977) Local regulation of adrenergic neurotransmission. Physiol Rev 57: 659-728

Presynaptic β-Adrenoceptors in Human Blood Vessels and Their Possible Relationship to Adenylate Cyclase

M. Göthert and F. Hentrich

Institut für Pharmakologie, Universitätsklinikum Essen, Hufelandstraße 55, 4300 Essen 1, Federal Republic of Germany

Presynaptic β-Adrenoceptors in Omental, Digital and Metatarsal Blood Vessels

Human blood vessels were used in one of the first attempts undertaken to clarify whether sympathetic nerve fibres are endowed with presynaptic β-adrenoceptors. In that study, Stjärne and Brundin (1975) demonstrated that in human omental arteries and veins (removed during surgery), adrenaline at low concentrations (up to 8 nmol/liter) and isoprenaline increased the electrically evoked ^{3}H-noradrenaline overflow. Propranolol, given alone, caused slight inhibition (less than 10%) of the evoked overflow; in interaction experiments, it abolished the facilitatory effect of isoprenaline (Stjärne and Brundin 1976).

In order to subclassify the presynaptic β-adrenoceptors, the authors applied agonists and antagonists that were rather subtype specific. Tazolol, a preferential β_1-adrenoceptor agonist, did not alter the evoked overflow, whereas the β_2-adrenoceptor agonists terbutaline and salbutamol had increasing effects. The facilitatory action of isoprenaline was abolished by the antagonist H 35/25, which exhibits a preference for β_2-adrenoceptors. However, it has not yet been shown whether propranolol (see above) or H 35/25 produced competitive antagonism, since in the interaction experiments only single concentrations of both the antagonists (1 µmol/liter) and isoprenaline (40 nmol/liter) were applied. The β_1-adrenoceptor antagonist practolol was ineffective in antagonizing the increasing effect of isoprenaline.

It was concluded that the β-adrenoceptors on the sympathetic nerve fibres of these blood vessels are of the β_2-subtype. In view of the limited ability of propranolol to inhibit release, when given alone, a positive β-adrenoceptor-mediated feedback control appeared to play, at best, a very small role. Rather, the data were compatible with a physiological significance of circulating adrenaline, which may activate these receptors (Stjärne and Brundin 1976).

Results in human digital arteries obtained at autopsy were equivocal concerning the subtype involved in β-adrenoceptor-mediated facilitation of electrically evoked ^{3}H-noradrenaline release. Thus, Stevens et al. (1982) reported that in these arteries, both the β_2-selective agonist salbutamol and the β_1-preferential agonist dobutamine (Wagner and Schümann 1979) increased ^{3}H-noradrenaline overflow. The authors did not conclude that presynaptic β_1- and β_2-adrenoceptors coexist on the sympathetic nerve fibres of this blood vessel. Rather they preferred to suggest that dobutamine is a non-selective agonist at the presynaptic β-adrenoceptors involved. Furthermore, they found that adrenaline 10 nmol/liter also caused facilitation. Propranolol, when given alone, did not affect the evoked release, whereas it abol-

New Aspects of the Role of Adrenoceptors in the Cardiovascular System/Ed. by Grobecker et al.

ished the facilitatory effects of salbutamol and adrenaline. Hence, there is clear-cut evidence for the conclusion that prejunctional β-adrenoceptors are present in human digital arteries (Stevens et al. 1982). Such receptors also appear to exist in human metatarsal veins, since salbutamol facilitated ^{3}H-noradrenaline release (Moulds and Stevens 1983). In this blood vessel as well, propranolol was ineffective when given alone. Here, interaction experiments with salbutamol were not carried out. In view of the failure of propranolol to decrease ^{3}H-noradrenaline release from both metatarsal veins and digital arteries, the authors concluded that presynaptic β-adrenoceptors are not activated by released noradrenaline (Moulds and Stevens, 1983). Since propranolol given alone also did not inhibit electrically evoked ^{3}H-noradrenaline release from digital arteries preincubated with a high concentration of unlabelled adrenaline (1 µmol/liter), it was suggested that released adrenaline, previously taken up into the neuronal storage sites, was not capable of stimulating these receptors. However, the possibility was considered that facilitatory presynaptic β-adrenoceptors may be activated under conditions of enhanced adrenomedullary secretion (Stevens et al. 1982).

Presynaptic β-Adrenoceptors in the Pulmonary Artery and Their Possible Relationship to Adenylate Cyclase

Controversial results as to the presence of presynaptic β-adrenoceptors have been obtained in pulmonary arteries of different animal species. Such receptors were identified in the guinea pig pulmonary artery (Misu et al. 1981, 1983), but they were not found in the rabbit pulmonary artery (Endo et al. 1977). In view of these discrepancies, we investigated whether facilitatory β-adrenoceptors are detectable on the sympathetic nerve fibres of the human pulmonary artery and, if present, to which subtype they belong (Göthert and Hentrich 1985).

The experiments were carried out on segments of human pulmonary arteries obtained from patients undergoing surgery for lung tumor. The segments were cut spirally into strips, which were incubated with ^{3}H-noradrenaline and then superfused with physiological salt solution (composition, see Göthert et al. 1984b) containing cocaine (30 µmol/liter) and corticosterone (40 µmol/liter). Three to five 3-min periods of transmural electrical stimulation (150 mA, 0.3 ms, 2 Hz) were applied at intervals of 24 min. Tritium efflux into the superfusate and tissue tritium were determined by liquid scintillation counting. The electrically evoked ^{3}H overflow (above basal efflux) was abolished by tetrodotoxin 1 µmol/liter or omission of calcium from the superfusion fluid. Separation of ^{3}H-noradrenaline from its ^{3}H-metabolites by combined use of alumina and Dowex columns (Graefe et al. 1973) revealed that 91% of the electrically evoked ^{3}H overflow was accounted for by unmetabolized ^{3}H-noradrenaline.

The electrically evoked ^{3}H-noradrenaline release was only slightly facilitated by prenalterol, an agonist with moderate preference for β_1-adrenoceptors, and it was strongly increased by isoprenaline and the selective β_2-adrenoceptor agonist procaterol (Fig. 1). Under identical conditions, adrenaline produced an inhibition of release (not shown), but after blockade of the presynaptic α-adrenoceptors with rau-

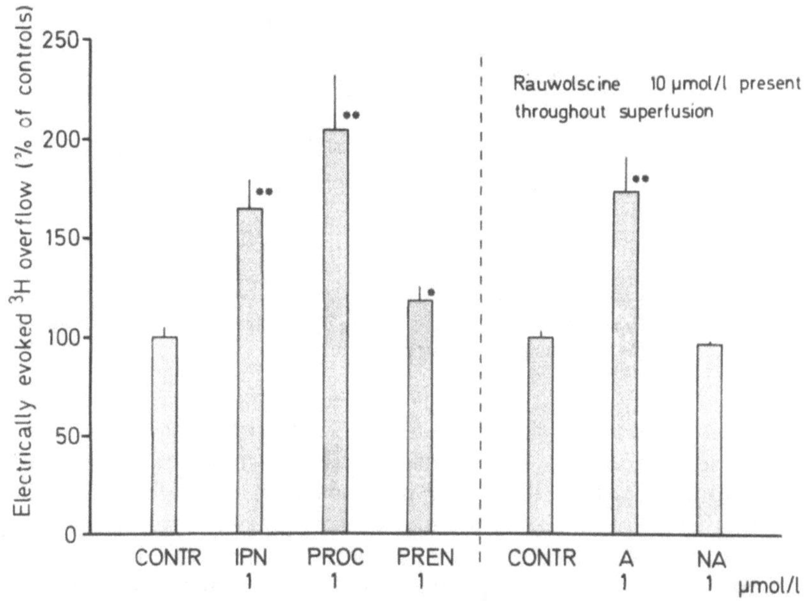

Fig. 1. Effects of adrenoceptor agonists (1 µmol/liter) on the electrically evoked ^3H overflow from strips of the human pulmonary artery. The strips were preincubated with ^3H-noradrenaline and superfused with physiological salt solution containing cocaine 30 µmol/liter plus corticosterone 40 µmol/liter (plus rauwolscine 10 µmol/liter in the experiments with adrenaline and noradrenaline; *right panel*). Five periods of transmural electrical stimulation (2 Hz, 3 min; S_1–S_5) at intervals of 24 min (S_1 after 93 min of superfusion). The ratios of the ^3H overflow evoked by S_5 to that evoked by S_2 are given (S_5/S_2). All ratios are expressed as percentages of the ratios in the control experiments *(CONTR)*. Each agonist was present 9 min before and during S_5. *IPN*, isoprenaline; *PROC*, procaterol; *PREN*, prenalterol; *A*, adrenaline; *NA*, noradrenaline. Means ± SEM of 4-6 experiments. $^*P < 0.05$; $^{**}P < 0.005$

wolscine, adrenaline caused a facilitation of release (Fig. 1). However, when noradrenaline was applied in the presence of rauwolscine, the evoked release was not affected (Fig. 1). In this context, it should be noted that, in contrast to adrenaline, which is an unselective agonist at β-adrenoceptors, noradrenaline exhibits a preference for the β_1-subtype.

The effects of β-adrenoceptor antagonists on the concentration-response curves of isoprenaline (0.01-1 µmol/liter; half-maximum facilitation of release at 95 nmol/liter) and of the β_2-selective agonist procaterol (0.01-1 µmol/liter; half-maximum facilitation at 63 nmol/liter) were also investigated (Table 1). The preferential β_2-adrenoceptor antagonist ICI 118-551 (Nahorski et al. 1979; Cook et al. 1984), but not the β_1-adrenoceptor antagonist atenolol, competitively antagonized the effect of procaterol. The facilitation of ^3H-noradrenaline release caused by isoprenaline was competitively antagonized by the unselective β-adrenoceptor antagonist propranolol, but not by atenolol (Table 1).

These results indicate that the sympathetic nerve fibres of the human pulmonary artery are endowed with facilitatory presynaptic β-adrenoceptors which belong to the β_2-subtype. When considering the inability of adrenaline - given alone - to in-

Table 1. Apparent pA_2 values of β-adrenoceptor antagonists for their antagonism against the facilitatory effect of isoprenaline or procaterol on the electrically evoked ^3H overflow from the human pulmonary artery preincubated with ^3H-noradrenaline

Antagonist	pA_2 value[a] against	
	Isoprenaline	Procaterol
Propranolol	7.96	Not determined
Atenolol	< 5.00[b]	< 5.00[b]
ICI 118-551	Not determined	7.99

[a] Determined from shifts to the right of the concentration-response curves of the agonists
[b] No shift to the right by atenolol 10 μmol/liter

crease and of propranolol to decrease the action potential-induced ^3H-noradrenaline release, it appears that the physiological importance of the facilitatory presynaptic β-adrenoceptors in the human pulmonary artery is rather small. Nevertheless, it is tempting to speculate that these receptors may play a role in the aetiopathology of certain diseases. Analogous to speculations concerning the role of presynaptic β-adrenoceptors in the development of systemic hypertension (Majewski 1983), it is conceivable that these receptors may be involved in the development of pulmonary hypertension.

It is well known that stimulation of β-adrenoceptors expresses its effect in a great variety of tissues via activation of an adenylate cyclase and the resulting increase in intracellular cyclic AMP (cAMP) respectively (Nathanson 1977). Therefore, the facilitation of noradrenaline release caused by β-adrenoceptor agonists may also be mediated by activation of an adenylate cyclase in the sympathetic nerves of the human pulmonary artery. However, the experimental approach to this problem must be very indirect, since sympathetic and other nerve fibres are embedded in tissue, largely composed of smooth muscle cells, which also contain an adenylate cyclase system. At present, no method is available for separating sympathetic nerve endings from smooth muscle cells and non-adrenergic nerve terminals. Therefore, direct analysis of intraneuronal cAMP and its modification by β-adrenoceptor agonists is not possible. In particular, it is impossible to investigate whether in sympathetic nerves a β-adrenoceptor-mediated increase in cAMP precedes the facilitation of noradrenaline release. However, in human pulmonary arteries, the question of whether drugs which presumably increase the intraneuronal cAMP concentration facilitate noradrenaline release and, hence, produce an effect which is identical to that of β-adrenoceptor agonists can be investigated (Hentrich et al. 1985).

For this purpose, forskolin, which activates adenylate cyclase by direct action on the catalytic subunit (Metzger and Lindner 1981; Seamon and Daly 1983), AH 21-132, which preferentially inhibits cAMP phosphodiesterase (Markstein et al. 1984) and the membrane-permeable cAMP analogue 8-Br-cAMP were applied. As summarized in Fig. 2, these compounds (concentration-dependently; not shown) increased the electrically evoked ^3H-noradrenaline release, and, hence, mimicked β-adrenoceptor agonists in this respect. Similar results were obtained in rabbit pulmonary arteries in which, however, the enzyme may be coupled to presynaptic adrenocorticotropic hormone (ACTH) receptors (Göthert and Hentrich 1984). The

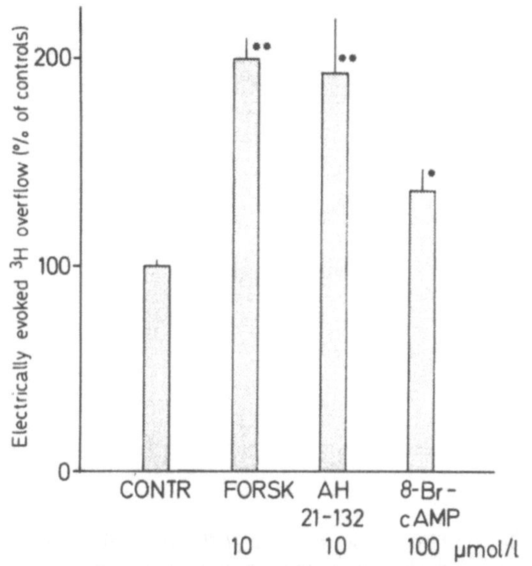

Fig. 2. Effects of forskolin *(FORSK)*, AH 21-132 (a phosphodiesterase inhibitor) and 8-bromo-adenosine 3′, 5′-cyclic monophosphate *(8-Br-cAMP)* on the electrically evoked ^3H overflow from strips of the human pulmonary artery. The strips were preincubated with ^3H-noradrenaline and superfused with physiological salt solution containing cocaine (30 µmol/liter) plus corticosterone (40 µmol/liter). Four periods of transmural electrical stimulation (2 Hz; S_1–S_4). The ratios S_4/S_2 are given (for further details, see legend to Fig. 1). Each compound was present 9 min before and during S_4. Means ± SEM of 6 or 7 experiments. $^*P < 0.01$; $^{**}P < 0.005$; *CONTR*, control

results obtained in these human or rabbit blood vessels suggest that the sympathetic nerve fibres contain adenylate cyclase and that cAMP may play a role in the regulation of action potential-induced noradrenaline release.

In order to obtain evidence of whether this adenylate cyclase may be coupled to presynaptic β-adrenoceptors, interaction experiments between forskolin and isoprenaline were carried out. Forskolin has been shown to potentiate the responses of cAMP generating systems to neurotransmitters and neuromodulators (Seamon and Daly 1983). The forskolin concentration of 0.3 µmol/liter applied in our interaction experiments produced only a rather small increase in evoked ^3H-noradrenaline release by itself (by about 35%; Hentrich et al. 1985). Isoprenaline 0.01 µmol/liter, when given alone, did not alter the electrically evoked ^3H overflow (Fig. 3). However, when forskolin 0.3 µmol/liter was present throughout superfusion, isoprenaline caused a clear-cut facilitation of release (Fig. 3). The concentration-response curve of isoprenaline (0.01–1 µmol/liter) was shifted to the left by forskolin 0.3 µmol/liter (Hentrich et al. 1985). These data are compatible with the involvement of adenylate cyclase in the facilitation of noradrenaline release caused by β-adrenoceptor activation.

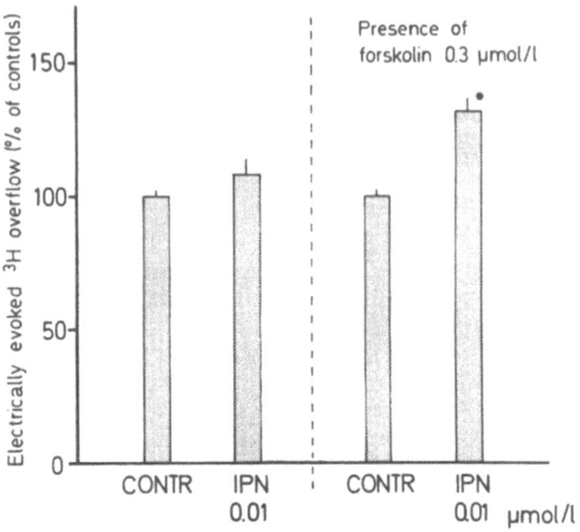

Fig. 3. Effect of isoprenaline *(IPN;* 10 nmol/liter) on the electrically evoked ^3H overflow from strips of the human pulmonary artery in the absence and presence of forskolin (*left and right panels*, respectively). The strips were preincubated with ^3H-noradrenaline and superfused with physiological salt solution containing cocaine (30 µmol/liter) plus corticosterone (40 µmol/liter). Three periods of transmural electrical stimulation (2 Hz; S_1–S_3) after 93, 117 and 141 min of superfusion. The ratios S_3/S_2 are given (for further details, see legend to Fig. 1). IPN was present 9 min before and during S_3; forskolin was added to the superfusion fluid from 9 min before S_2 until the end of the experiments. *CONTR*, controls. Means ± SEM of 5 or 6 experiments. $^*P < 0.001$

Presynaptic β-Adrenoceptors in the Saphenous Vein and Their Functional Interplay with Other Adrenoceptors in the Synapse

Presynaptic β-adrenoceptors on the sympathetic nerve fibres are also found in the human saphenous vein. This conclusion may be drawn from the experiments shown in Fig. 4 which were for the most part carried out under the same conditions as those in the experiments on human pulmonary artery (the slight difference in the time schedule of electrical stimulation is indicated in the legend). The electrically evoked ^3H overflow was facilitated by adrenaline (in the presence of rauwolscine) and isoprenaline. Propranolol, when given alone, did not significantly alter the evoked ^3H overflow, but at a concentration of 0.1 µmol/liter, it competitively antagonized the facilitatory effect of isoprenaline (data not shown; for similar results, see Verbeuren et al. 1983). A differentiation of the β-adrenoceptor subtype involved has not yet been carried out, but in analogy to the β-adrenoceptors in the other human blood vessels, it may be assumed that they belong to the β_2-subtype.

The pattern of adrenoceptors in the synapse between a sympathetic nerve fibre and a smooth muscle cell is illustrated in Fig. 5. Released or exogenously applied noradrenaline activates three different adrenoceptors, namely inhibitory presynaptic α_2-adrenoceptors (Janssens and Verhaeghe 1983; Göthert et al. 1984), which are involved in fine regulation of noradrenaline release, and postsynaptic α_1- and α_2-adrenoceptors (Zerkowski et al. 1984), which mediate the contraction of vascular

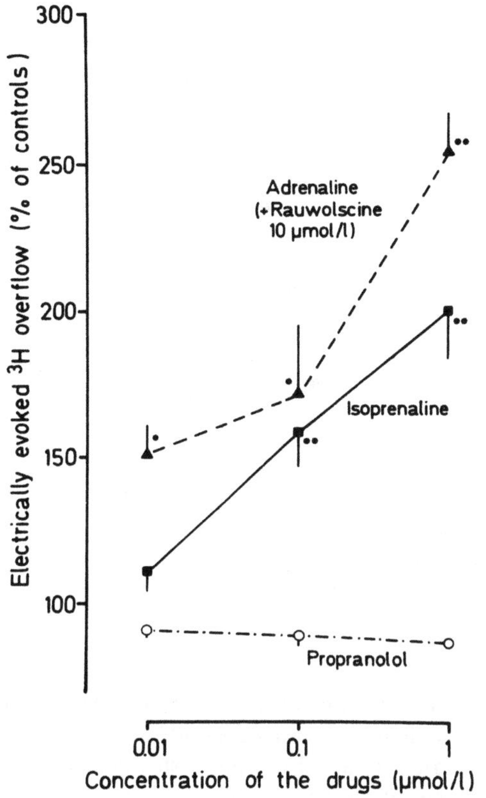

Fig. 4. Effects of adrenaline, isoprenaline and propranolol on the electrically evoked ^3H overflow from strips of the human saphenous vein. The strips were preincubated with ^3H-noradrenaline and superfused with physiological salt solution containing cocaine 30 μmol/liter plus corticosterone 40 μmol/l (plus rauwolscine 10 μmol/liter in the experiments with adrenaline). Five periods of transmural electrical stimulation (2 Hz, 3 min; S_1–S_5) at intervals of 32 min (S_1 after 94 min of superfusion; for further details of methods, see Göthert et al., 1984). The ratios of the ^3H overflow evoked by S_3, S_4 and S_5 to that evoked by S_2 are given. All ratios are expressed as percentages of the ratios in the control experiments. Each concentration of the drugs (▲, adrenaline; ■, isoprenaline; ○, propranolol) was present 12 min before and during the stimulation period S_3, S_4 or S_5. Means ± SEM of 4–5 experiments. $*P<0.05$, $**P<0.005$ (compared with the corresponding controls)

smooth muscle. The effect of adrenaline is even more complex, since this agonist stimulates not only these three receptors, but also pre- and postsynaptic β-adrenoceptors. Isoprenaline activates "only" two receptors, namely the pre- and postsynaptic β-adrenoceptors, leading to a facilitation of noradrenaline release and a direct relaxation of vascular smooth muscle respectively (Verbeuren et al. 1983).

The complex interplay between the functionally synergistic and antagonistic effects has not yet been investigated thoroughly. Only one study exists in which the influence of isoprenaline on the contraction evoked by exogenous noradrenaline or by electrical stimulation of the sympathetic nerves contained in strips of the human saphenous vein was analysed (Verbeuren et al. 1983). Isoprenaline, by activating postsynaptic β-adrenoceptors, produced a slight relaxation of strips previously con-

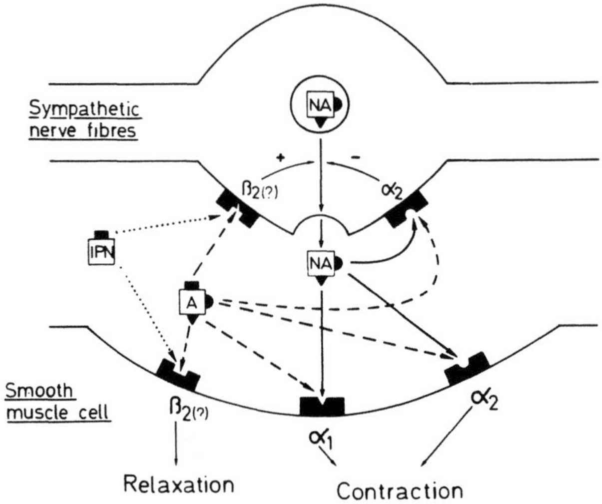

Fig. 5. Schematic representation of pre- and postsynaptic adrenoceptors in the human saphenous vein and the effects mediated by them. The scheme is based on the results shown in Fig. 4 and on those of Verbeuren et al. (1983), Zerkowski et al. (1984) and Göthert et al. (1984). *A*, adrenaline; *NA*, noradrenaline; *IPN*, isoprenaline; +, facilitation of release; −, inhibition of release

tracted by exogenous noradrenaline. Transmural electrical stimulation of the sympathetic nerves caused a contraction of smooth muscle, which in turn was mediated via an activation of the postsynaptic α-adrenoceptors by released noradrenaline. When, in addition, isoprenaline was administered, an increase in evoked ^{3}H-noradrenaline overflow and in the contractile response to nerve stimulation was observed. The increased contraction occurred despite of the weak relaxing effect of isoprenaline mediated by the postsynaptic β-adrenoceptors (see above) and is obviously caused by the increased concentration of endogenous noradrenaline at the postsynaptic α-adrenoceptors. Hence, in the human saphenous vein, the functional importance of the presynaptic β-adrenoceptors predominates over that of the postsynaptic β-adrenoceptors (the opposite was observed in canine saphenous veins; Verbeuren et al. 1983).

Functional Importance of Presynaptic β-Adrenoceptors

It can be concluded from the previous section that complex interplay with the various adrenoceptors is important for the maintenance of blood vessel normal function. An impairment of the physiological equilibrium, e.g., by changes of the number or "sensitivity" of β-adrenoceptors, may play a role in the pathogenesis of certain diseases. Thus, it has been suggested that presynaptic β-adrenoceptors in heart and blood vessels may be involved in the development of essential hypertension (Lokhandwala and Eickenburg 1983; Majewski 1983). Increased β-adrenoceptor-mediated facilitation of noradrenaline release by adrenaline may occur in this disease (Majewski 1983) or in pulmonary hypertension. However, at present, no data obtained in blood vessels from hypertensive patients are available which could support the hypothesis that presynaptic β-adrenoceptors may be altered in hypertension.

Summary

The sympathetic nerve fibres of various human blood vessels (omental arteries and veins, digital arteries, metatarsal veins, saphenous vein and pulmonary artery) are endowed with presynaptic β-adrenoceptors. Activation of these receptors by, e.g., isoprenaline increases action potential-induced noradrenaline release, and this effect is competitively antagonized by propranolol.

In pulmonary artery and omental blood vessels, the β-adrenoceptor subtype involved was determined by means of subtype-selective agonists and antagonists. It was found that the presynaptic β-adrenoceptors are of the β_2-subtype. Accordingly, the natural transmitter noradrenaline, which preferentially activates β_1-receptors (in addition to its activation of α-adrenoceptors) did not increase noradrenaline release, even when the presynaptic α_2-adrenoceptors were blocked by rauwolscine.

In omental blood vessels and digital arteries, low concentrations of adrenaline facilitated the evoked noradrenaline release, suggesting that the presynaptic β-adrenoceptors may be activated by circulating adrenaline under conditions of enhanced adrenomedullary secretion. At present, there is little evidence for the possibility that released adrenaline, previously taken up from the circulation into the neuronal storage sites, may exert a positive β-adrenoceptor-mediated feedback control of noradrenaline release, since propranolol produced a slight inhibition of release only in omental arteries and veins and not in the other blood vessels investigated.

Although the physiological importance of presynaptic β-adrenoceptors may be rather small, they may play a considerable role in the aethiopathology of certain diseases, such as systemic and pulmonary hypertension.

References

Cook N, Richardson A, Barnett DB (1984) Comparison of the β_1 selective affinity of prenalterol and corwin demonstrated by radioligand binding. Eur J Pharmacol 98: 407-412

Endo T, Starke K, Bangerter A, Taube HD (1977) Presynaptic receptor systems on the noradrenergic neurones of the rabbit pulmonary artery. Naunyn-Schmiedebergs Arch Pharmacol 296: 229-247

Göthert M, Hentrich F (1984) Role of cAMP for regulation of impulse-evoked noradrenaline release from the rabbit pulmonary artery and its possible relationship to presynaptic ACTH receptors. Naunyn Schmiedebergs Arch Pharmacol 328: 127-134

Göthert M, Hentrich F (1985) Identification of presynaptic β_2-adrenoceptors on the sympathetic nerve fibres of the human pulmonary artery. Br J Pharmacol 85: 933-941

Göthert M, Schlicker E, Hentrich F, Rohm N, Zerkowski HR (1984) Modulation of noradrenaline release in human saphenous vein via presynaptic α_2-adrenoceptors. Eur J Pharmacol 102: 261-267

Graefe KH, Stefano FJE, Langer SZ (1973) Preferential metabolism of (–)-^{3}H-norepinephrine through the deaminated glycol in the rat vas deferens. Biochem Pharmacol 22: 1147–1160
Hentrich F, Göthert M, Greschuchna D (1985) Involvement of cAMP in modulation of noradrenaline release in the human pulmonary artery. Naunyn-Schmiedebergs Arch Pharmacol 330: 245–247
Janssens W, Verhaeghe R (1983) Modulation of the concentration of noradrenaline at neuro-effector junction in human saphenous vein. Br J Pharmacol 79: 577–585
Lokhandwala MF, Eikenburg DC (1983) Presynaptic receptors and alterations in norepinephrine release in spontaneously hypertensive rats. Life Sci 33: 1527–1542
Majewski H (1983) Modulation of noradrenaline release through activation of presynaptic β-adrenoreceptors. J Auton Pharmacol 3: 47–60
Markstein R, Digges K, Marshall NR, Starke K (1984) Forskolin and the release of noradrenaline in cerebrocortical slices. Naunyn-Schmiedebergs Arch Pharmacol 325: 17–24
Metzger H, Lindner E (1981) The positive inotropic-acting forskolin, a potent adenylate cyclase activator. Arzneimittelforsch/Drug Res 31: 1248–1250
Misu Y, Kaiho M, Ogawa K, Kubo T (1981) Adrenergic transmission failure via the blockade of presynaptic beta receptors in guinea-pig pulmonary arteries. J Pharmacol Exp Ther 218: 242–247
Misu Y, Kuwahara M, Kaiho M, Kubo T (1983) Further characterization of presynaptic β-adrenoceptors in guinea-pig pulmonary arteries. Eur J Pharmacol 91: 287–290
Moulds RFW, Stevens MJ (1983) Facilitatory prejunctional β-adrenoceptors in human arteries and veins. Gen Pharmacol 14: 81–83
Nahorski SR, Howlett DR, Redgrave P (1979) Loss of β-adrenoceptor binding sites in rat striatum following kainic acid lesions. Eur J Pharmacol 60: 249–252
Nathanson JA (1977) Cyclic nucleotides and nervous system function. Physiol Rev 57: 157–256
Seamon KB, Daly JW (1983) Forskolin, cyclic AMP and cellular physiology. Trends Pharmacol Sci 4: 120–123
Stevens MJ, Rittinghausen RE, Medcalf RL, Moulds RFW (1982) Prejunctional β-adrenoceptors in human digital arteries. Eur J Pharmacol 83: 263–270
Stjärne L, Brundin J (1975) Dual adrenoceptor-mediated control of noradrenaline secretion from human vasoconstrictor nerves: facilitation by β-receptors and inhibition by α-receptors. Acta Physiol Scand 94: 139–141
Stjärne L, Brundin J (1976) β_2-Adrenoceptors facilitating noradrenaline secretion from human vasoconstrictor nerves. Acta Physiol Scand 97: 88–93
Verbeuren TJ, Lorenz RR, Aarhus LL, Shepherd JT, Vanhoutte PM (1983) Prejunctional beta-adrenoceptors in human and canine saphenous veins. J Auton Nerv Syst 8: 261–271
Wagner J, Schümann HJ (1979) Stimulation of β-adrenoceptors by dobutamine in the guinea-pig atrium and tracheal chain. Naunyn-Schmiedebergs Arch Pharmacol 308: 19–23
Zerkowski HR, Wagner J, Rohm N, Rodrigues-Pereira E, Reidemeister JC (1984) Postsynaptic alpha$_1$- and alpha$_2$-adrenoceptor subtypes in the human saphenous vein. Blood Vessels 21: 147

In Vivo Operation of Prejunctional Adrenoceptors in the Peripheral Sympathetic Nervous System

K. Starke, H. Majewski, H. Ensinger, B. Szabo, and L. Hedler

Pharmakologisches Institut, Universität Freiburg, Hermann-Herder-Straße 5, 7800 Freiburg i. Br., Federal Republic of Germany

Introduction

In his review on the electrophysiology of postganglionic sympathetic neurones which was published in 1972, Haefely included a chapter entitled "Adrenoceptors of the Adrenergic Neuron". He pointed out that adrenoceptors had been identified only in sympathetic ganglia; there was no evidence for their existence at axons or axon terminals. It is noteworthy that this picture has changed entirely. It is now clear that terminal noradrenergic axons, both in the central nervous system and in the periphery, do possess adrenoceptors, in fact, all three major types: α-adrenoceptors, β-adrenoceptors and dopamine receptors. The function that is modified when these prejunctional receptors are activated is the action potential-evoked release of noradrenaline. Activation of α-adrenoceptors and dopamine receptors decreases the release per action potential, whereas activation of β-adrenoceptors leads to an increase. Much more is known today about prejunctional adrenoceptors than about the receptors occurring in sympathetic ganglia (for review, see Langer 1977, 1981; Starke 1977, 1981a; Gillespie 1980; Rand et al. 1980).

Even today, however, an important gap in our knowledge concerns the operation of prejunctional adrenoceptors in vivo. By far the majority of studies have been carried out on isolated tissues. The main reason is most likely the difficulty involved in assessing in vivo the release of noradrenaline per action potential. We summarize here experiments that were designed to study prejunctional adrenoceptors at peripheral sympathetic neurones of the rabbit in vivo. The "noradrenaline spillover rate" was determined in order to estimate the overall peripheral release of noradrenaline.

The Model

The basic procedure was to determine not only the plasma noradrenaline level, but also the rate of clearance of noradrenaline from the plasma. From these two parameters, and given steady-state conditions, the *rate at which neuronally released noradrenaline enters plasma,* called here the *noradrenaline spillover rate,* can be calculated as the product of the plasma level of noradrenaline and the plasma noradrenaline clearance. Plasma noradrenaline clearance was measured by intravenous infusion of a tracer dose of (–)-^{3}H-noradrenaline until a steady-state plasma concentration was reached. The plasma noradrenaline clearance then equals the ra-

New Aspects of the Role of Adrenoceptors in the Cardiovascular System/Ed. by Grobecker et al.

tio of the ^{3}H-noradrenaline infusion rate to the steady-state plasma ^{3}H-noradrenaline concentration. It is emphasized that the noradrenaline spillover rate is the rate at which transmitter enters into plasma and not the rate at which it is released from the sum of all peripheral noradrenergic neurones. The total neuronal release cannot be determined at present. However, the noradrenaline spillover rate is an index of neuronal release and is a better index than the plasma noradrenaline level alone because the removal of noradrenaline from the plasma is taken into account. For instance, in both humans (Esler et al. 1981) and anaesthetized rabbits (Majewski et al. 1982), blockade of neuronal noradrenaline uptake by desipramine did not change the plasma noradrenaline level, but decreased noradrenaline clearance from the plasma. From these findings a reduced spillover rate is calculated, indicating that desipramine in fact decreased neuronal release of noradrenaline, despite the unchanged plasma level. In the studies summarized below, yohimbine and its diastereomer rauwolscine increased the plasma noradrenaline level. However, this was only partly due to an increased release from the neurones, because at the same time, the plasma noradrenaline clearance was decreased. Calculation of the noradrenaline spillover rate yielded a more appropriate estimate of the alkaloid-induced increase in neuronal release. The measurement of noradrenaline kinetics in vivo is discussed in a recent review article by Esler et al. (1984).

The rabbits were either anaesthetized with pentobarbitone, pithed, pithed and nephrectomized, or conscious. In pithed rabbits, the sympathetic outflow was continuously stimulated by electrical pulses delivered at 2 or 3 Hz via the pithing rod. Blood for the determination of noradrenaline and ^{3}H-noradrenaline was sampled from a femoral or carotid artery. Noradrenaline was determined by high-pressure liquid chromatography followed by electrochemical detection. ^{3}H-Noradrenaline was separated from its metabolites by column chromatography and quantified by liquid scintillation counting. Since a tracer dose was infused, ^{3}H-noradrenaline did not contribute to the plasma level of (endogenous) noradrenaline. All parameters were measured three times (P_1, P_2, P_3) and only after the plasma ^{3}H-noradrenaline concentration had stabilized. The times of measurement differed in the various experimental series, with P_1 at 50–110 min after the onset of ^{3}H-noradrenaline infusion, P_2 20–30 min after P_1 and P_3 20–30 min after P_2. All drugs were given intravenously immediately after P_1 as bolus injections and/or infusions. Values read at P_2 and P_3 were expressed as a percentage of P_1.

In the following discussion, only those two parameters are presented that are most relevant to the subject, i.e., mean arterial pressure and the noradrenaline spillover rate. For details, the reader is referred to the original reports (Majewski et al. 1983a–c, 1984; Schmidt et al. 1984; Ensinger et al. 1985).

Prejunctional Dopamine Receptors

Studies on isolated tissues indicate that many, but not all, peripheral noradrenergic neurones possess prejunctional dopamine receptors, the activation of which inhibits action potential-evoked release of noradrenaline. In our in vivo experiments, the ergot derivative bromocriptine and the 1-phenyl-3-benzazepine fenoldopam (SKF 82526) were used as agonists. Domperidone and (R)-(+)-8-chloro-2,3,4,5-tetrahydro-3-methyl-5-phenyl-1H-3-benzazepin-7-ol (SCH 23390) were used as antagonists.

Bromocriptine diminished the plasma noradrenaline level in anaesthetized rabbits, and Fig. 1 shows that this was due to a decrease in the noradrenaline spillover rate and coincided with a fall in mean arterial pressure. Each parameter was reduced to a similar degree at P_2 and P_3 (30 and 60 min after P_1 respectively). The DA_1-receptor-selective antagonist SCH 23390 failed to counteract bromocriptine, but both effects of the agonist were abolished by the DA_2-receptor-selective antagonist domperidone (for selectivities, see Hilditch and Drew 1985). The findings indicate that bromocriptine decreases noradrenaline release and thereby reduces blood pressure by activation of DA_2-receptors, without a detectable contribution of DA_1-receptors. Moreover, antagonism by domperidone suggests that the DA_2-receptors involved occur in the periphery, since domperidone does not readily cross the blood-brain barrier (Laduron and Leysen 1979).

In order to substantiate a peripheral site of action, further experiments were carried out in rabbits in which the central nervous system was destroyed by pithing and the sympathetic outflow stimulated electrically at a constant frequency. Figure 2 shows that under these conditions bromocriptine lowered blood pressure and the noradrenaline spillover rate. The percentage decrease was at least as high as in anaesthetized rabbits. Again, the effect of bromocriptine was prevented by domperidone.

The effect of the second dopamine receptor agonist used, i.e. fenoldopam, differed markedly from the effect of bromocriptine (Fig. 3). Although fenoldopam also decreased mean arterial pressure in pithed rabbits with electrically stimulated sym-

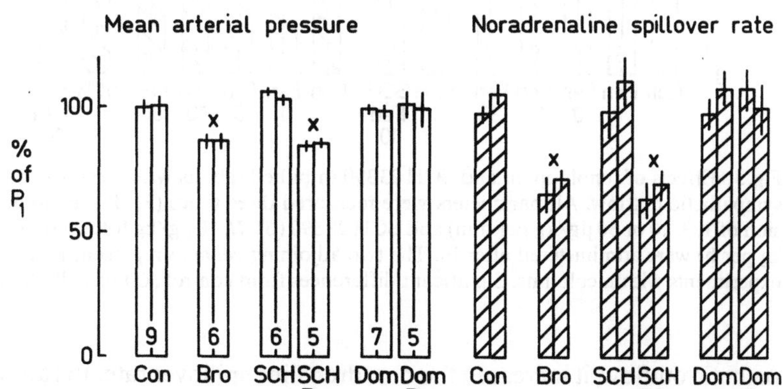

Fig. 1. Effects of bromocriptine, SCH 23390 and domperidone in anaesthetized rabbits. All parameters were measured three times (P_1–P_3). Bromocriptine (*Bro*, 40 μg/kg infused over 20 min), SCH 23390 (*SCH*, 10 μg/kg followed by infusion of 2 μg/kg per h) and domperidone (*Dom*, 200 μg/kg followed by infusion of 50 μg/kg per h) were administered after P_1. The two adjoining *columns* represent P_2 and P_3. Numbers of experiments within columns. Significant differences from control *(Con)*: *x*, $P<0.05$. Modified from Ensinger et al. (1985)

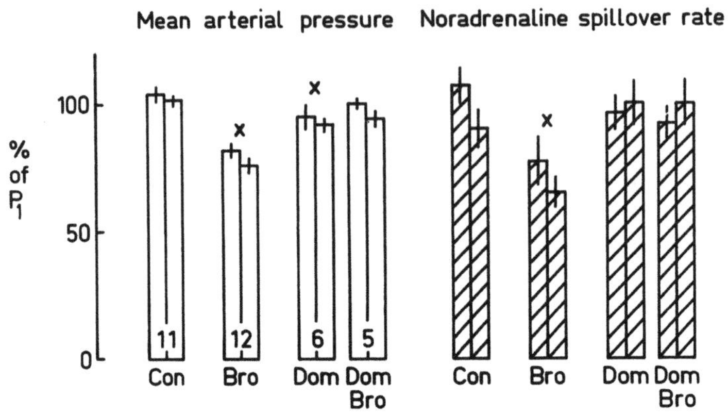

Fig. 2. Effects of bromocriptine and domperidone in pithed rabbits with electrically stimulated (2 Hz) sympathetic outflow. All parameters were measured three times (P_1–P_3). Bromocriptine (*Bro*, 40 μg/kg infused over 20 min) and domperidone (*Dom*, 200 μg/kg followed by infusion of 50 μg/kg per h) were administered after P_1. The two adjoining *columns* represent P_2 and P_3. Numbers of experiments within columns. Significant differences from control *(Con)*: *x*, $P<0.05$. Modified from Ensinger et al. (1985)

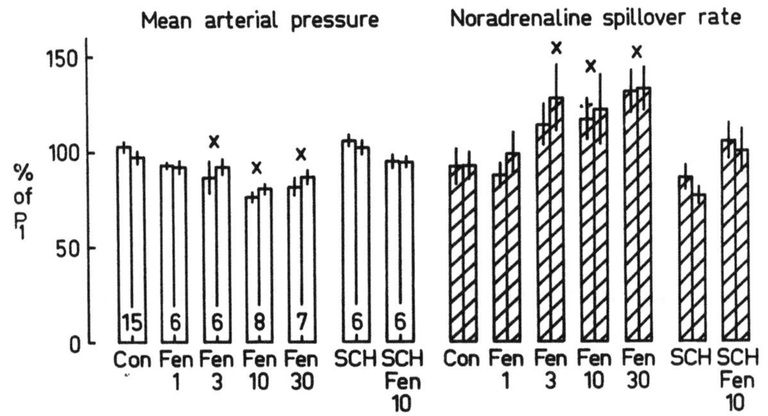

Fig. 3. Effects of fenoldopam and SCH 23390 in pithed rabbits with electrically stimulated (2 Hz) sympathetic outflow. All parameters were measured three times (P_1–P_3). Fenoldopam (*Fen*, infusion of 1, 3, 10 or 30 μg/kg per min) and SCH 23390 (*SCH*, 10 μg/kg followed by infusion of 2 μg/kg per h) were administered after P_1. The two adjoining *columns* represent P_2 and P_3. Numbers of experiments within columns. Significant differences from control *(Con)*: *x*, $P<0.05$.

pathetic outflow, it increased the noradrenaline spillover rate. In further contrast, its hypotensive effect was antagonized by the same dose of SCH 23390 that failed to antagonize bromocriptine. Since fenoldopam is a DA_1-selective agonist (see Lokhandwala et al. 1985), these observations further support the view that the prejunctional inhibitory dopamine receptors are exclusively DA_2. The decrease in blood pressure elicited by fenoldopam presumably reflects the activation of postjunctional, vasodilation-mediating vascular DA_1-receptors. We do not know the reason for the increase in the noradrenaline spillover rate; one possibility would be blockade of prejunctional α_2-adrenoceptors (Foley and Sarau 1984) and, hence, interruption of the α_2-adrenergic autoinhibition of noradrenaline release (see below).

Our experiments are compatible with the operation of prejunctional DA_2-receptors at postganglionic sympathetic neurones in vivo. They are in accordance with the majority of reports indicating that bromocriptine lowers the plasma noradrenaline concentration (e.g. Mannelli et al. 1984; see, however, Nagahama et al. 1984) and demonstrate that this reflects a decreased spillover into plasma rather than an increased removal from the plasma. In agreement with our findings in rabbits, the ergot derivative pergolide reduced the plasma noradrenaline level in pithed rats with electrically-stimulated sympathetic outflow (Cavero et al. 1984). Dopamine itself also activates prejunctional dopamine receptors in anaesthetized rabbits (Ensinger et al. 1985). It should be noted that domperidone, when given alone, did not change the noradrenaline spillover rate (Figs. 1 and 2). This supports the prevailing opinion (see Gillespie 1980; Rand et al. 1980; Langer 1981) that prejunctional dopamine receptors, although they can be activated by exogenous agonists, normally do not receive an endogenous input.

Prejunctional β-Adrenoceptors

Studies in vitro indicate that many, but not all, postganglionic sympathetic axon terminals possess β-adrenoceptors, the activation of which enhances action potential-evoked release of noradrenaline. In their original description of prejunctional β-adrenoceptors, Adler-Graschinski and Langer (1975) suggested that these receptors might serve a physiological role in that endogenous noradrenaline activated them and, hence, facilitated its own release. In view of the great potential significance of such positive feedback, the small number of in vivo investigations is particularly surprising.

Infusion of isoprenaline in anaesthetized rabbits increased the plasma noradrenaline level. Figure 4 shows that this was due to an increase in the noradrenaline spillover rate and coincided with a decrease in mean arterial pressure. For each parameter, the changes at P_2 and P_3 (30 and 60 min after P_1, respectively) were similar. A fall in blood pressure will per se enhance the release of noradrenaline via the baroreceptor reflex. However, the directly acting vasodilator drug hydralazine at an equihypotensive dose increased the noradrenaline spillover rate much less than did isoprenaline ($P<0.05$). The β_2-selective antagonist erythro-(±)-1-(7-methylindan-4-yloxy)-3-isopropylaminobutan-2-ol (ICI 118551; Bilski et al. 1983) abolished both the (β_2-adrenergic) hypotension and the increase in spillover rate caused by isoprenaline (Fig. 4) but did not affect the (β_1-adrenergic) isoprenaline-induced tachycardia (not shown). Furthermore, the β_1-selective antagonist atenolol failed to counteract the effect of isoprenaline on noradrenaline spillover (not shown). These findings indicate that isoprenaline increases noradrenaline release more than can be explained by the blood pressure fall and that the receptor involved is of the β_2-type.

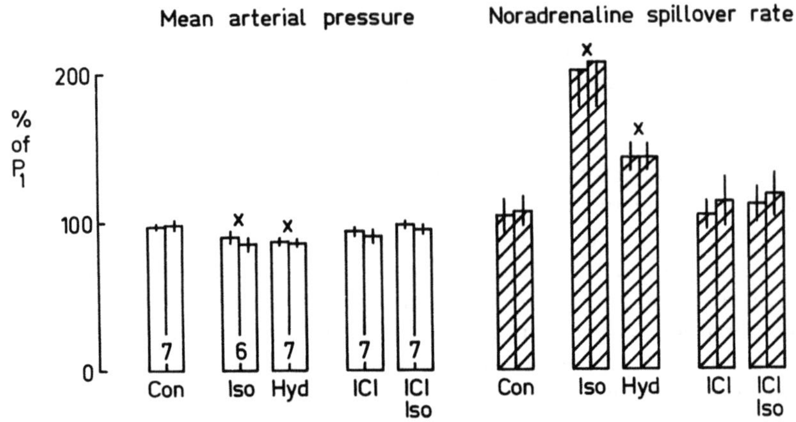

Fig. 4. Effects of isoprenaline, hydralazine and ICI 118551 in anaesthetized rabbits. All parameters were measured three times (P_1–P_3). Isoprenaline (*Iso*, infusion of 0.5 µg/kg per min), hydralazine (*Hyd*, 0.2 mg/kg) and ICI 118551 (*ICI*, 0.3 mg/kg followed by infusion of 0.1 mg/kg per h) were administered after P_1. The two adjoining *columns* represent P_2 and P_3. Numbers of experiments within columns. Significant differences from control *(Con): x*, $P<0.05$. Modified from Schmidt et al. (1984)

Activation of β-adrenoceptors at the renal juxtaglomerular cells elicits renin secretion; in the rabbit, the receptors are β_2 (Keeton and Campbell 1981). Angiotensin II prejunctionally facilitates the release of noradrenaline from many peripheral neurones (see Starke 1977; Langer 1981). An infusion of angiotensin II in fact enhanced the noradrenaline spillover rate in pithed nephrectomized rabbits with electrically stimulated sympathetic outflow (Majewski et al. 1984). It seemed possible, therefore, that isoprenaline increased noradrenaline release, not directly at prejunctional β-adrenoceptors, but indirectly via the kidney and the renin-angiotensin system. In order to test this possibility, isoprenaline 0.5 µg/kg per min was administered to pithed nephrectomized rabbits with electrically stimulated sympathetic outflow. The persistence of the increase in noradrenaline spillover under these conditions (Schmidt et al. 1984) indicates that the effect is largely independent of the kidney. Moreover, the observation demonstrates that β-adrenergic facilitation does not require an intact central nervous system.

Our experiments correspond to the operation of prejunctional β-adrenoceptors at postganglionic sympathetic neurones in vivo. Graded infusions of isoprenaline in humans cause graded increases in the plasma noradrenaline level. Although a more complete analysis must be restricted to animal experiments, the observation suggests that the prejunctional β-receptor mechanism can be activated by exogenous agonists in humans as well (Vincent et al. 1982). Moreover, in rabbits as in humans (Vincent et al. 1984), the receptors seem to be β_2, a view that is consistent with most in vitro work (see Gillespie 1980; Rand et al. 1980; Langer 1981; Majewski 1983). It should be noted that ICI 118551, when given alone, did not change the noradrenaline spillover rate (Fig. 4). Apparently, prejunctional β-adrenoceptors are not activated by an endogenous compound under these conditions. In one of the earliest in vivo studies on prejunctional adrenoceptors, Yamaguchi et al. (1977) showed that isoprenaline increased and, conversely, that the β-antagonist sotalol decreased the overflow of noradrenaline into the coronary sinus elicited by cardio-accelerator nerve stimulation in dogs. Similarly, propranolol and metoprolol diminished the electrically evoked venous overflow of noradrenaline from cat and dog skeletal muscle (Dahlöf 1981). More recent experiments by Cousineau et al. (1984) indicate, however, that the effect of sotalol may have been due to an increased inactivation of noradrenaline within the cardiac tissue rather than to decreased neuronal release. The prevailing evidence today tends to disagree with the view that prejunctional β-adrenoceptors normally mediate a positive feedback mechanism facilitating the release of noradrenaline. It has been suggested that positive feedback may develop when the potent β_2-agonist adrenaline, rather than the weak β_2-agonist noradrenaline, activates prejunctional β_2-receptors (see Majewski 1983; Osswald and Guimarães 1983).

Prejunctional α-Adrenoceptors

Work on isolated tissues has established beyond a doubt that almost all peripheral noradrenergic terminal axons possess α-adrenoceptors. Their activation depresses action potential-evoked release of noradrenaline. It is widely accepted that the receptors are physiological action sites of neuronally released noradrenaline and, hence, "autoreceptors" that mediate a negative feedback mechanism. Studies on prejunctional α-adrenoceptors led to the distinction of two major pharmacological subtypes of α-receptors, α_1 and α_2 (see Starke 1981 b). The prejunctional receptors were the prototype α_2-adrenoceptors, and it seems likely that, although there may also be some prejunctional α_1-adrenoceptors, the latter are a minority. In our experiments , yohimbine and rauwolscine were used as selective α_2-antagonists and corynanthine and prazosin as selective α_1-antagonists. The antagonists were given at subtype-selective doses. For studies of the release-inhibiting effect of α-adrenoceptor agonists in conscious and pithed rabbits, the reader is referred to the original publications (Majewski et al. 1983 a, b).

Initial experiments were carried out in conscious rabbits. As shown in Fig. 5, corynanthine did not change, whereas the α_2-selective compounds yohimbine and rauwolscine increased mean arterial pressure and the noradrenaline spillover rate. On the one hand, these results are compatible with the operation of prejunctional α-adrenoceptors in conscious rabbits, as well as with the receptors' α_2-properties and their relay function in a negative feedback mechanism. On the other hand, alternative explanations are obvious. Yohimbine-like alkaloids, in particular yohimbine itself and rauwolscine, can cause behavioural excitation (see Goldberg and Robertson 1983) and an increase in sympathetic nervous discharge (McCall et al. 1983). Hence, yohimbine and rauwolscine may have acted primarily on the central nervous system, increasing the firing rate of the sympathetic neurones and, consequently, noradrenaline release and blood pressure.

Central sympatho-excitatory effects of the yohimbine alkaloids are less pronounced after anaesthesia (Rockhold and Gross 1981). Therefore, we next investi-

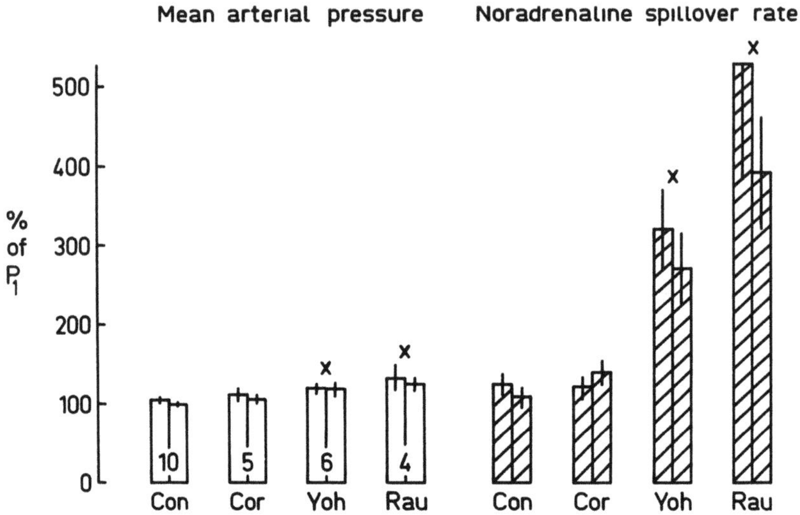

Fig. 5. Effects of corynanthine, yohimbine and rauwolscine in conscious rabbits. All parameters were measured three times (P_1–P_3). Corynanthine (*Cor,* 1 mg/kg), yohimbine (*Yoh,* 1 mg/kg) and rauwolscine (*Rau,* 1 mg/kg) were administered after P_1. The two adjoining *columns* represent P_2 and P_3. Numbers of experiments within columns. Significant differences from control *(Con): x,* $P <$ 0.05. Modified from Majewski et al. (1983 a)

gated the effects of α-adrenoceptor antagonists in anaesthetized rabbits. Rauwolscine, corynanthine and prazosin lowered blood pressure under these conditions (Figs. 6, 7). In order to take into account a possible reflex acceleration of sympathetic firing, it was necessary, as in the case of isoprenaline, to administer directly acting vasodilators for comparison. The drugs chosen were hydralazine and sodium nitroprusside. From all vasodilator experiments, groups were formed in which the fall in arterial pressure matched the fall produced by a given α-antagonist. Figure 6 shows that yohimbine increased the noradrenaline spillover rate despite unchanged blood pressure. Moreover, rauwolscine caused a slight decrease in blood pressure, and only rauwolscine and not the equihypotensive vasodilators increased the noradrenaline spillover. The α_1-selective antagonists elicited an entirely different pattern of effects. They reduced mean arterial pressure more markedly than rauwolscine (Fig. 7). Yet, whereas the vasodilators caused a pronounced increase in noradrenaline spillover, no increase was obtained with corynanthine and 0.3 mg/kg prazosin. In each case, the noradrenaline spillover rate upon administration of the α_1-antagonist was significantly *lower* than upon administration of equihypotensive vasodilators ($P <$ 0.05). The results are again consistent with the operation and autoreceptor function of prejunctional α_2-adrenoceptors in the rabbit in vivo. The apparent dampening, by corynanthine and prazosin, of the baroreceptor-mediated increase in noradrenaline release is of interest, although not directly related to the present subject. It indicates that α_1-antagonists, in addition to blocking peripheral α_1-adrenoceptors, depress the activation of the sympathetic nervous system in response to a fall in blood pressure, possibly via a central site of action (see Majewski et al. 1983 c).

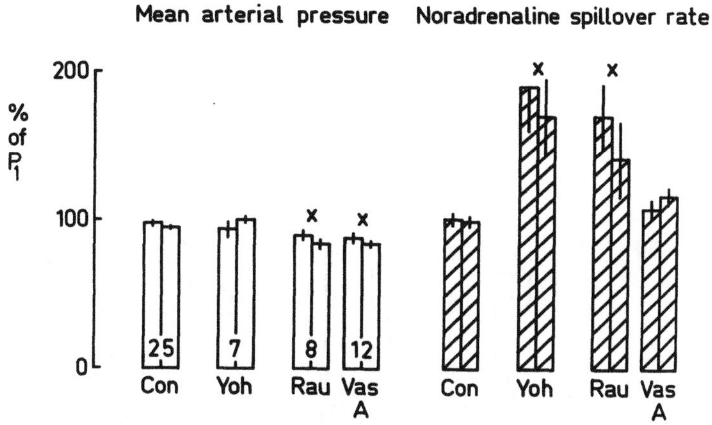

Fig. 6. Effects of yohimbine and rauwolscine in anaesthetized rabbits. All parameters were measured three times (P_1-P_3). Yohimbine (*Yoh*, 1 mg/kg) and rauwolscine (*Rau*, 1 mg/kg) were administered after P_1. For comparison with rauwolscine, the effects in an equihypotensive vasodilator group are shown, composed of experiments with hydralazine (0.1-1.25 mg/kg) and sodium nitroprusside (infusion of 1-10 μg/kg per min) which were also administered after P_1 *(Vas A)*. The two adjoining *columns* represent P_2 and P_3. Numbers of experiments within columns. Significant differences from control *(Con)*: *x*, $P < 0.05$. Modified from Majewski et al. (1983c)

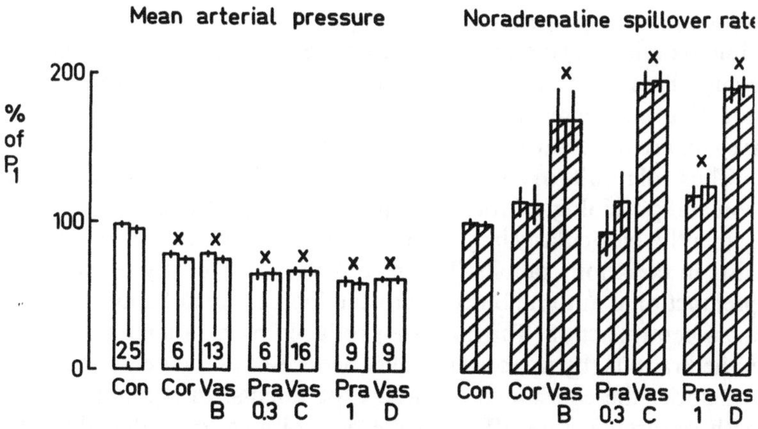

Fig. 7. Effects of corynanthine and prazosin in anaesthetized rabbits. All parameters were measured three times (P_1-P_3). Corynanthine (*Cor*, 1 mg/kg) and prazosin (*Pra*, 0.3 or 1 mg/kg) were administered after P_1. For comparison with corynanthine and the two doses of prazosin, the effects in equihypotensive vasodilator groups are shown, composed of experiments with hydralazine (0.1-1.25 mg/kg) and sodium nitroprusside (infusion of 1-10 μg/kg per min) which were also administered after P_1 *(Vas B, Vas C* and *Vas D)*. The two adjoining *columns* represent P_2 and P_3. Numbers of experiments within columns. Significant differences from control *(Con)*: *x*, $P < 0.05$. Modified from Majewski et al. (1983c)

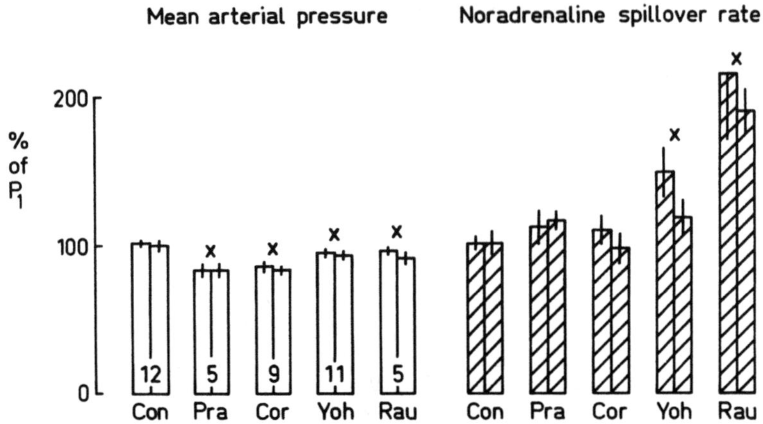

Fig. 8. Effects of prazosin, corynanthine, yohimbine and rauwolscine in pithed rabbits with electrically stimulated (3 Hz) sympathetic outflow. All parameters were measured three times (P_1–P_3). Prazosin (*Pra*, 0.1 mg/kg), corynanthine (*Cor*, 1 mg/kg), yohimbine (*Yoh*, 1 mg/kg) and rauwolscine (*Rau*, 1 mg/kg) were administered after P_1. The two adjoining columns represent P_2 and P_3. Numbers of experiments within columns. Significant differences from control *(Con): x*, $P < 0.05$. Modified from Majewski et al. (1983b)

A final series of experiments was carried out in pithed rabbits with electrically stimulated sympathetic outflow. Figure 8 shows that prazosin, corynanthine, yohimbine and rauwolscine all lowered mean arterial pressure. Only the α_2-selective compounds increased the noradrenaline spillover rate. α_1-Selective compounds did not effect any increase. The results, obtained after destruction of the central nervous system, are in accordance with the α_2-autoreceptor hypothesis.

Thus, all results in conscious, anaesthetized and pithed rabbits support the operation and physiological role of prejunctional α_2-adrenoceptors in vivo. It seems likely that the particularly large increase in noradrenaline release caused by α_2-antagonists in conscious rabbits (by up to 400%) only partly reflects the interruption of prejunctional autoinhibition, with the increase also being brought about by a primary central action. The increase produced by α_2-antagonists in anaesthetized and pithed rabbits (by up to 100%) may better reveal the degree of autoinhibition existing under the conditions of these experiments. In previous in vivo studies, drugs with α-adrenoceptor affinity have been shown to modify the venous overflow of noradrenaline from tissues upon sympathetic nerve stimulation or exercise, as predicted by the autoreceptor hypothesis (Yamaguchi et al. 1977; Cavero et al. 1979; Yamaguchi 1982; Cousineau et al. 1984; Heyndrickx et al. 1984; see also the article that paved the way for the detection of prejunctional α-adrenoceptors: Brown and Gillespie 1957). In addition, such drugs modify as predicted the plasma noradrenaline concentration in man (Elliott et al. 1984), as well as in conscious or anaesthetized animals or pithed animals with electrically stimulated sympathetic outflow (Graham et al. 1980; Yamaguchi and Kopin 1980; Saeed et al. 1982; see, however, Hamilton et al. 1982) and the tissue noradrenaline content (Wakade and Wakade 1984). The effect of α-adrenoceptor antagonists on the noradrenaline spillover rate has not been investigated previously, and although the α_2-agonist clonidine reduces the noradrenaline spillover rate in humans (see Esler et al. 1984), this is mainly a central nervous effect.

General Comment

In the intact rabbit, all three adrenoceptors previously demonstrated in isolated tissues appear to operate. They are activated by appropriate agonists, blocked by appropriate antagonists and mediate the expected response. They belong, for the most part, to the DA_2-, β_2- and α_2-subtypes, respectively. Only the α_2-receptors seem to be autoreceptors, i. e., normal targets of the neurone's own transmitter.

A non-prejunctional location of the release-modulating receptors that has not been excluded in our experiments is in sympathetic ganglia. This reservation holds true not only for the conscious and anaesthetized rabbit, but also for the pithed rabbit, since electrical stimulation as used here is predominantly preganglionic (Majewski et al. 1984). Inhibitory dopamine receptors and α-adrenoceptors, as well as facilitatory β-adrenoceptors, occur in some sympathetic ganglia (see Haefely 1972; Cavero et al. 1982). However, the number of ganglia in which such receptors have been described is small, in contrast to the wide distribution of prejunctional adrenoceptors. Moreover, all pharmacological properties of the receptors found in vivo agree very well with the characteristics established for prejunctional adrenoceptors in vitro in ganglion-free preparations. It has been suggested that ganglionic dopamine receptors are of the DA_1-subtype (Grega et al. 1984). If this were true, the DA_2-character of the release-inhibiting dopamine receptors in anaesthetized and pithed rabbits would rule out a ganglionic location. While the involvement of prejunctional adrenoceptors in the results obtained seems definite, a contribution from ganglionic sites remains an interesting, yet somewhat speculative, possibility.

Terminal axons of postganglionic sympathetic neurones possess a variety of receptors, in addition to adrenoceptors and receptors for angiotensin II. We have recently shown that ethylketocyclazocine decreases the noradrenaline spillover rate in pithed rabbits with electrically stimulated sympathetic outflow via a prejunctional opioid receptor (Ensinger et al. 1984). Determination of the noradrenaline spillover rate in anaesthetized, conscious and pithed rabbits lends itself to further study of prejunctional receptor systems under quasi-physiological conditions.

Summary

Experiments on isolated tissues have shown that terminal postganglionic sympathetic axons possess α-adrenoceptors, β-adrenoceptors and dopamine receptors. We have studied these receptors in anaesthetized, pithed and conscious rabbits. From the plasma noradrenaline concentration and the clearance of noradrenaline from the plasma, the rate of entry into plasma, i. e., the noradrenaline spillover rate, was calculated. The dopamine receptor agonist bromocriptine decreased the spillover rate. Its effect was prevented by the DA_2-selective antagonist domperidone, but not by the DA_1-selective antagonist SCH 23390. In contrast to bromocriptine, the DA_1-selective agonist fenoldopam increased the spillover rate. When given alone, domperidone caused no change. Isoprenaline increased the spillover rate more than was accounted for by the fall in blood pressure. Its effect was blocked by the β_2-selective antagonist ICI 118551, which, when given alone, caused no change. The noradrenaline spillover rate was increased by the α_2-selective antagonists yohimbine and rauwolscine, but not by the α_1-selective antagonists corynanthine and prazosin. These findings indicate that, in vivo as well as in vitro, the release of noradrenaline per action potential can be inhibited via prejunctional α_2- and DA_2-receptors and facilitated via prejunctional β_2-receptors. Only the α_2-adrenoceptors appear to be normal targets of released noradrenaline itself.

References

Adler-Graschinsky E, Langer SZ (1975) Possible role of a β-adrenoceptor in the regulation of noradrenaline release by nerve stimulation through a positive feed-back mechanism. Br J Pharmacol 53: 43-50

Bilski AJ, Halliday SE, Fitzgerald JD, Wale JL (1983) The pharmacology of a β_2-selective adrenoceptor antagonist (ICI 118,551). J Cardiovasc Pharmacol 5: 430-437

Brown GL, Gillespie JS (1957) The output of sympathetic transmitter from the spleen of the cat. J Physiol (Lond) 138: 81-102

Cavero I, Dennis T, Lefèvre-Borg F, Perrot P, Roach AG, Scatton B (1979) Effects of clonidine, prazosin and phentolamine on heart rate and coronary sinus catecholamine concentration during cardioaccelerator nerve stimulation in spinal dogs. Br J Pharmacol 67: 283-292

Cavero I, Massingham R, Lefèvre-Borg F (1982) Peripheral dopamine receptors, potential targets for a new class of antihypertensive agents. Life Sci 31: 1059-1069

Cavero I, Lefèvre-Borg F, Lhoste F, Sabatier C, Richer C, Giudicelli JF (1984) Pharmacological, hemodynamic and autonomic nervous system mechanisms responsible for the blood pressure and heart rate lowering effects of pergolide in rats. J Pharmacol Exp Ther 228: 779-791

Cousineau D, Goresky CA, Bach GG, Rose CP (1984) Effect of β-adrenergic blockade on in vivo norepinephrine release in canine heart. Am J Physiol 246: H283-H292

Dahlöf C (1981) Studies on β-adrenoceptor mediated facilitation of sympathetic neurotransmission. Acta Physiol Scand 114, Suppl 500

Elliott HL, Jones CR, Vincent J, Lawrie CB, Reid JL (1984) The alpha adrenoceptor antagonist properties of idazoxan in normal subjects. Clin Pharmacol Ther 36: 190-196

Ensinger H, Hedler L, Schurr C, Starke K (1984) Ethylketocyclazocine decreases noradrenaline release and blood pressure in the rabbit at a peripheral opioid receptor. Naunyn-Schmiedebergs Arch Pharmacol 328: 20-23

Ensinger H, Majewski H, Hedler L, Starke K (1985) Neuronal and postjunctional components in the blood pressure effects of dopamine and bromocriptine in rabbits. J Pharmacol Exp Ther 234: 681-690

Esler M, Jackman G, Leonard P, Skews H, Bobik A, Korner P (1981) Effect of norepinephrine uptake blockers on norepinephrine kinetics. Clin Pharmacol Ther 29: 12-20

Esler M, Jennings G, Korner P, Blomberry P, Sacharias N, Leonard P (1984) Measurement of total and organ-specific norepinephrine kinetics in humans. Am J Physiol 247: E21-E28

Foley JJ, Sarau HM (1984) Adrenergic binding studies of SK&F 82526 and its enantiomers. Fed Proc 43: 555

Gillespie JS (1980) Presynaptic receptors in the autonomic nervous system. In: Szekeres L (ed) Adrenergic activators and inhibitors, part I. Springer, Berlin Heidelberg New York, pp 353-425 (Handbook of experimental pharmacology, vol 54/I)

Goldberg MR, Robertson D (1983) Yohimbine: a pharmacological probe for study of the α_2-adrenoceptor. Pharmacol Rev 35: 143-180

Graham RM, Stephenson WH, Pettinger WA (1980) Pharmacological evidence for a functional role of the prejunctional alpha-adrenoceptor in noradrenergic neurotransmission in the conscious rat. Naunyn-Schmiedebergs Arch Pharmacol 311: 129-138

Grega GJ, Barrett RJ, Adamski SW, Lokhandwala MF (1984) Effects of dopamine (DA) and SKF 82526, a selective DA_1-receptor agonist, on vascular resistances in the canine forelimb. J Pharmacol Exp Ther 229: 756-762

Haefely W (1972) Electrophysiology of the adrenergic neuron. In: Blaschko H, Muscholl E (eds) Catecholamines. Springer, Berlin Heidelberg New York, pp 661-725 (Handbook of experimental pharmacology, vol 33)

Hamilton CA, Reid JL, Zamboulis C (1982) The role of presynaptic α-adrenoceptors in the regulation of blood pressure in the conscious rabbit. Br J Pharmacol 75: 417-424

Heyndrickx GR, Vilaine JP, Moerman EJ, Leusen I (1984) Role of prejunctional α_2-adrenergic receptors in the regulation of myocardial performance during exercise in conscious dogs. Circ Res 54: 683-693

Hilditch A, Drew GM (1985) Peripheral dopamine receptor blockade by SCH 23390 and domperidone in vitro. Eur J Pharmacol 116: 171-174

Keeton TK, Campbell WB (1981) The pharmacologic alteration of renin release. Pharmacol Rev 32: 81-227

Laduron PM, Leysen JE (1979) Domperidone, a specific in vitro dopamine antagonist, devoid of in vivo central dopaminergic activity. Biochem Pharmacol 28: 2161-2165

Langer SZ (1977) Presynaptic receptors and their role in the regulation of transmitter release. Br J Pharmacol 60: 481-497

Langer SZ (1981) Presynaptic regulation of the release of catecholamines. Pharmacol Rev 32: 337-362

Lokhandwala MF, Watkins HO, Sabouni MH, Alkadhi KA (1985) Pharmacological analysis of the actions of SKF 82526 on cardiovascular dopamine receptors. J Pharmacol Exp Ther 234: 337-344

Majewski H (1983) Modulation of noradrenaline release through activation of presynaptic β-adrenoreceptors. J Auton Pharmacol 3: 47-60

Majewski H, Hedler L, Starke K (1982) The noradrenaline release rate in the anaesthetized rabbit: facilitation by adrenaline. Naunyn-Schmiedebergs Arch Pharmacol 321: 20-27

Majewski H, Hedler L, Starke K (1983 a) Modulation of noradrenaline release in the conscious rabbit through α-adrenoceptors. Eur J Pharmacol 93: 255-264

Majewski H, Hedler L, Starke K (1983 b) Evidence for a physiological role of presynaptic α-adrenoceptors: modulation of noradrenaline release in the pithed rabbit. Naunyn-Schmiedebergs Arch Pharmacol 324: 256-263

Majewski H, Rump LC, Hedler L, Starke K (1983 c) Effects of α_1- and α_2-adrenoceptor blocking drugs on noradrenaline release rate in anaesthetized rabbits. J Cardiovasc Pharmacol 5: 703-711

Majewski H, Hedler L, Schurr C, Starke K (1984) Modulation of noradrenaline release in the pithed rabbit: a role for angiotensin II. J Cardiovasc Pharmacol 6: 888-896

Mannelli M, Delitala G, de Feo ML, Maggi M, Cuomo S, Piazzini M, Guazzelli R, Serio M (1984) Effects of different dopaminergic antagonists on bromocriptine-induced inhibition of norepinephrine release. J Clin Endocrinol Metab 59: 74-78

McCall RB, Schuette MR, Humphrey SJ, Lahti RA, Barsuhn C (1983) Evidence for a central sympathoexcitatory action of alpha-2 adrenergic antagonists. J Pharmacol Exp Ther 224: 501-507

Nagahama S, Chen Y, Oparil S (1984) Mechanism of the depressor effect of bromocriptine in the spontaneously hypertensive rat. J Pharmacol Exp Ther 228: 370-375

Osswald W, Guimarães S (1983) Adrenergic mechanisms in blood vessels: morphological and pharmacological aspects. Rev Physiol Biochem Pharmacol 96: 53-122

Rand MJ, McCulloch MW, Story DF (1980) Catecholamine receptors on nerve terminals. In: Szekeres L (ed) Adrenergic activators and inhibitors. Springer, Berlin Heidelberg New York, pp 223-266 (Handbook of experimental pharmacology, vol 54/I)

Rockhold RW, Gross F (1981) Yohimbine diastereoisomers: cardiovascular effects after central and peripheral application in the rat. Naunyn-Schmiedebergs Arch Pharmacol 315: 227-231

Saeed M, Sommer O, Holtz J, Bassenge E (1982) α-Adrenoceptor blockade by phentolamine causes β-adrenergic vasodilation by increased catecholamine release due to presynaptic α-blockade. J Cardiovasc Pharmacol 4: 44-52

Schmidt HHHW, Schurr C, Hedler L, Majewski H (1984) Local modulation of noradrenaline release in vivo: presynaptic β_2-adrenoceptors and endogenous adrenaline. J Cardiovasc Pharmacol 6: 641-649
Starke K (1977) Regulation of noradrenaline release by presynaptic receptor systems. Rev Physiol Biochem Pharmacol 77: 1-124
Starke K (1981 a) Presynaptic receptors. Ann Rev Pharmacol 21: 7-30
Starke K (1981 b) α-Adrenoceptor subclassification. Rev Physiol Biochem Pharmacol 88: 199-236
Vincent HH, Man in't Veld AJ, Boomsma F, Wenting GJ, Schalekamp MADH (1982) Elevated plasma noradrenaline in response to β-adrenoceptor stimulation in man. Br J Clin Pharmacol 13: 717-721
Vincent HH, Boomsma F, Man in't Veld AJ, Derkx FHM, Wenting GJ, Schalekamp MADH (1984) Effects of selective and non-selective β-agonists on plasma potassium and norepinephrine. J Cardiovasc Pharmacol 6: 107-114
Wakade AR, Wakade TD (1984) Reduction in norepinephrine content of sympathetic neuroeffector organs by alpha adrenergic antagonists and nerve stimulation: evidence for presynaptic control of sympathetic transmitter release in intact animal. J Pharmacol Exp Ther 228: 287-292
Yamaguchi I, Kopin IJ (1980) Differential inhibition of alpha-1 and alpha-2 adrenoceptor-mediated pressor responses in pithed rats. J Pharmacol Exp Ther 214: 275-281
Yamaguchi N (1982) Evidence supporting the existence of presynaptic α-adrenoceptors in the regulation of endogenous noradrenaline release upon hepatic sympathetic nerve stimulation in the dog liver in vivo. Naunyn-Schmiedebergs Arch Pharmacol 321: 177-184
Yamaguchi N, de Champlain J, Nadeau RA (1977) Regulation of norepinephrine release from cardiac sympathetic fibers in the dog by presynaptic α- and β-receptors. Circ Res 41: 108-117

Transmitter Coexistence in the Sympathetic Nervous System: Impact on Cardiovascular Regulation

H. Grobecker

Lehrstuhl für Pharmakologie, Universität Regensburg, Universitätsstraße 31, 8400 Regensburg, Federal Republic of Germany

In recent years, evidence has been obtained for ATP and noradrenaline as cotransmitters in sympathetic nerves (cf. Burnstock and Sneddon 1985). The existence and storage of ATP together with noradrenaline in vesicles of sympathetic nerves was first reported by Schümann (1958). The author found that ATP and noradrenaline were stored in the vesicles in a molar ratio of 1 to 4. In the past decade, coexistence situations in sympathetic neurones have been described both for classical transmitters, such as noradrenaline and adrenaline, and for the coexistence of catecholamines and peptides (Hökfelt et al. 1980, Rand et al. 1983). These results are of interest in the context of changes in adrenoceptor-catecholamine interactions, e. g. in the development of high blood pressure in both experimental and human essential hypertension, and may have also implications for the therapeutic action of β-receptor blocking drugs in essential hypertension.

Adrenaline as a Cotransmitter in Essential Hypertension in Man

In investigations by our laboratory, we have reported elevated plasma catecholamines (noradrenaline and adrenaline) in young hypertensive and hyperkinetic patients (Dominiak and Grobecker, 1982). Plasma catecholamine concentrations are considered to be reliable indices of sympatho-neuronal (noradrenaline) and sympatho-adrenal (adrenaline) activity and reactivity in man. Clinically, hypertensive patients were characterized by elevated systolic and diastolic blood pressure and increased heart rate, whereas patients with hyperkinetic heart syndrome had increased heart rate and increased systolic blood pressure, while diastolic blood pressure was normal (Fig. 1 a, b). At rest, there was a significant positive correlation between heart rate and circulating catecholamines in both groups of patients. In hypertensives, a positive correlation between heart rate and plasma adrenaline concentrations could be observed, while patients with hyperkinetic heart syndrome presented positive correlation between heart rate and plasma noradrenaline concentrations. Sympatho-neuronal and sympatho-adrenal reactivity during mental stress or physical exercise increased in both groups of patients, mirrored by an increase in blood pressure and heart rate. Pindolol is a potent non-selective β-adrenoceptor blocking drug with intrinsic sympathomimetic activity and minimal membrane stabilizing properties. When administered in a single oral dose of 10 mg, pindolol diminished the exaggerated sympathetic tone in both groups of patients by attenuating circulating catecholamine levels at rest or during mental stress, but not during physical exercise (Fig. 2 a, b).

New Aspects of the Role of Adrenoceptors in the Cardiovascular System/Ed. by Grobecker et al.

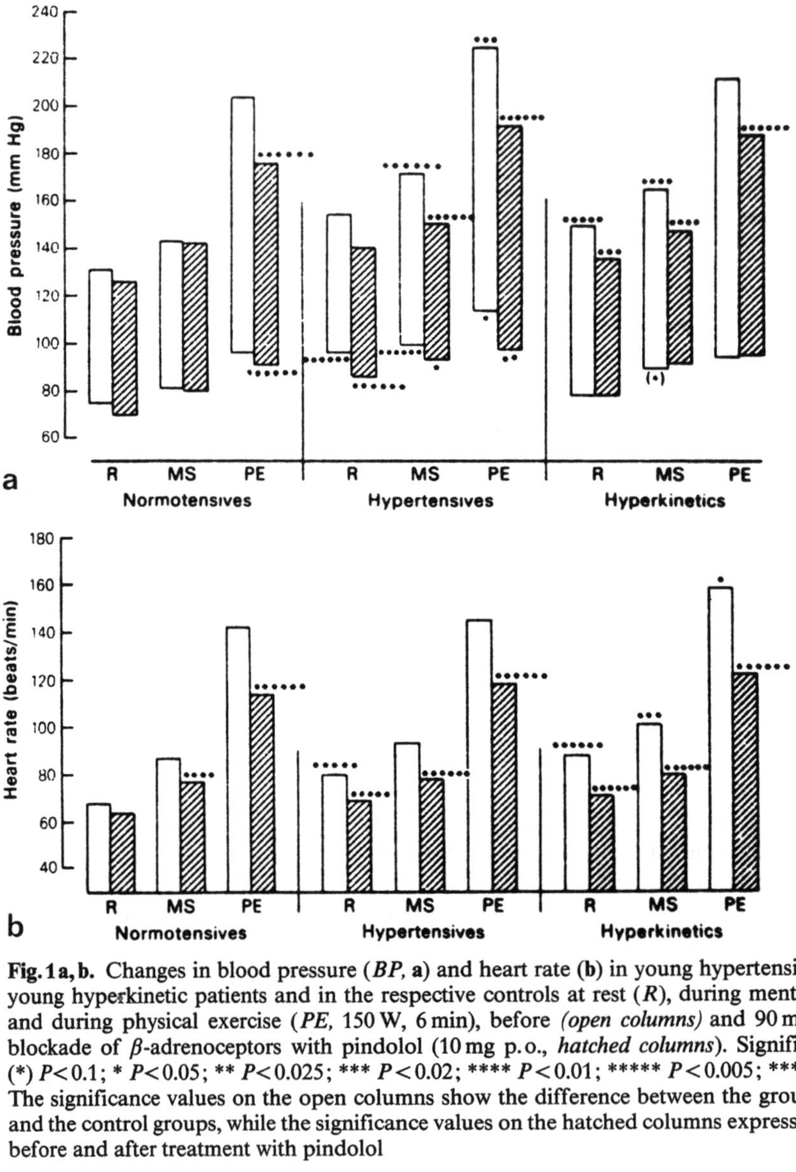

Fig. 1 a, b. Changes in blood pressure (*BP*, **a**) and heart rate (**b**) in young hypertensive patients, in young hyperkinetic patients and in the respective controls at rest (*R*), during mental stress (*MS*) and during physical exercise (*PE*, 150 W, 6 min), before *(open columns)* and 90 min after acute blockade of β-adrenoceptors with pindolol (10 mg p.o., *hatched columns*). Significance (*t* test): (*) $P<0.1$; * $P<0.05$; ** $P<0.025$; *** $P<0.02$; **** $P<0.01$; ***** $P<0.005$; ****** $P<0.001$. The significance values on the open columns show the difference between the groups of patients and the control groups, while the significance values on the hatched columns express the difference before and after treatment with pindolol

From these results it is concluded that β-adrenoceptor blocking drugs such as pindolol may exert their anti-hypertensive activity partially by blockade of prejunctional β-adrenoceptors (Fig. 3).

Recently, the role of adrenaline in essential hypertension in man was also described by Brown (1984). The author reported that adrenaline (0.05 µg/kg per min i.v.) was able to elevate plasma noradrenaline concentrations in volunteers significantly when presynaptic α-receptors were blocked by idazoxan (0.2 mg/kg), a specific α_2-receptor antagonist. Adrenaline infusion in the same subjects after adminis-

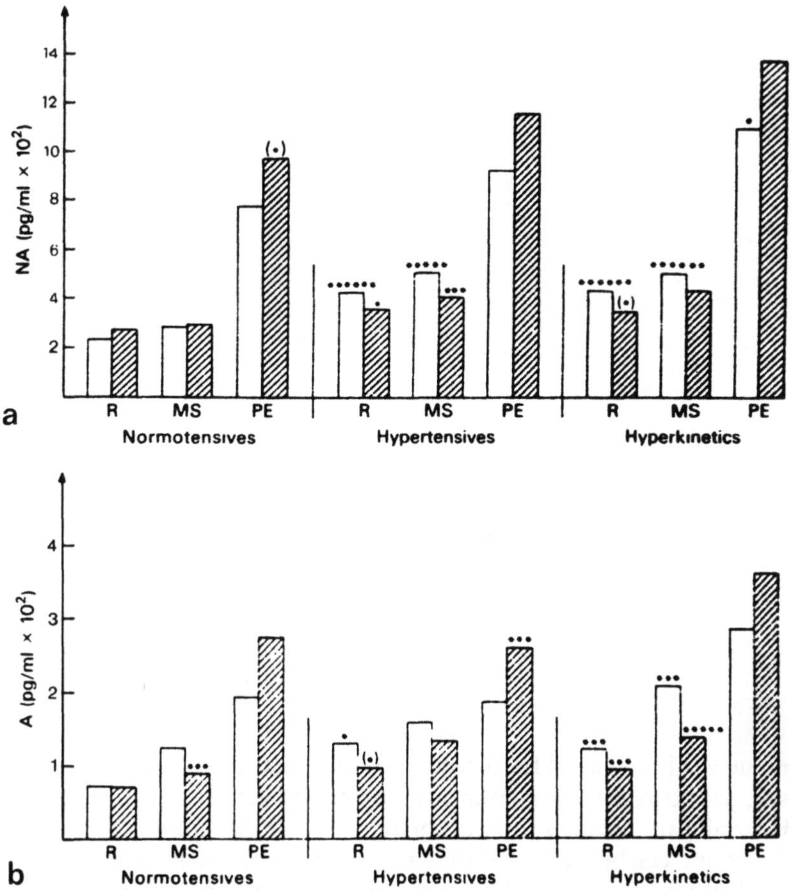

Fig. 2 a, b. Changes in plasma noradrenaline (**a**) and adrenaline concentrations (**b**) in young hypertensive patients, in young hyperkinetic patients and in the respective controls at rest (*R*), during mental stress (*MS*) and during physical exercise (*PE*, 150 W, 6 min) before *(open columns)* and 90 min after acute blockade of β-adrenoceptors with pindolol (10 mg p.o., *hatched columns*). Significance (*t* test): see Fig. 1 a

tration of placebo was without effect on plasma noradrenaline, because adrenaline then simultaneously activated presynaptic facilitatory β_2- and presynaptic inhibitory α_2-adrenoceptors and because the latter action presumably balanced the former.

Transmitter-Peptide Coexistence in Peripheral Sympathetic Neurones

In the past 4 years, the occurrence of both classical transmitters and peptides in the same neurones of peripheral nerves and the central nervous system have been demonstrated by the immunohistochemical technique (cf. Hökfelt et al. 1980). This tech-

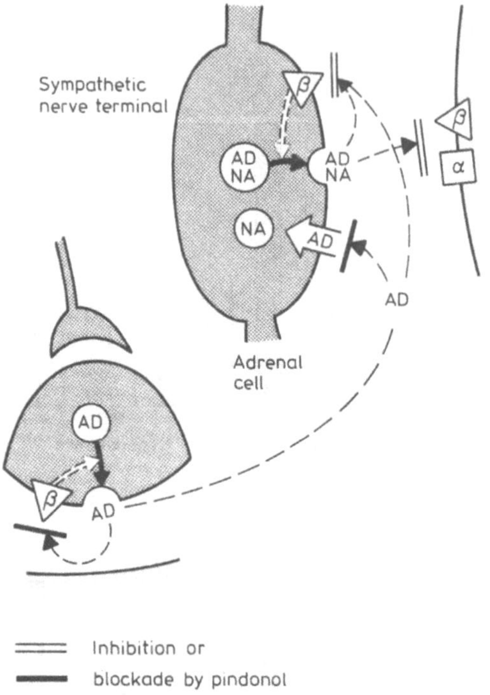

Fig. 3. Presynaptic inhibition of noradrenaline (*NA*) release by pindolol. The possible function of adrenaline (*AD*) as a cotransmitter is depicted

nique has been useful for detection of different types of compounds in nervous tissue, provided that the substances are immunogenic (or can be made immunogenic by conjugation with a carrier protein) and that the substances are available in pure forms and can be retained during processing for immunohistochemistry (for details, see Hökfelt et al. 1980). However, several limitations of the immunohistochemical method must be discussed. An evident problem is the specificity of the immunological reaction. Furthermore, the method may not be sensitive enough to detect very small amounts of the peptides, or the relatively large antibody molecules may not easily be able to penetrate intracellular storage sites.

These complex conditions have caused divergent views on, e.g. the occurrence and distribution of the opioid peptides in peripheral and central neurones, described first by Hughes et al. (1975) as pentapeptides Leu- and Met-enkephalin. Later, Larsson et al. (1979) described separate neurones for Leu- and Met-enkephalin. Moreover, the distribution of β-endorphin in neurones of the central nervous system remains to be established. Sometimes the administration of colchicine or nerve ligation are helpful methods for accumulating the peptides in the axoplasm before immunocytochemical mapping is done.

According to Hökfelt et al. (1980), a peptidergic neurone can be characterized schematically as shown in Fig. 4, although up to now only a limited amount of information has been available. Like the well-known peripheral adrenergic neurones, peptide neurones also possess large granular vesicles. However, in contrast to the adrenergic neurones, there is no local synthesis of the transmitter. Peptides are probably produced only on the ribosomes of the cell soma as precursor molecules.

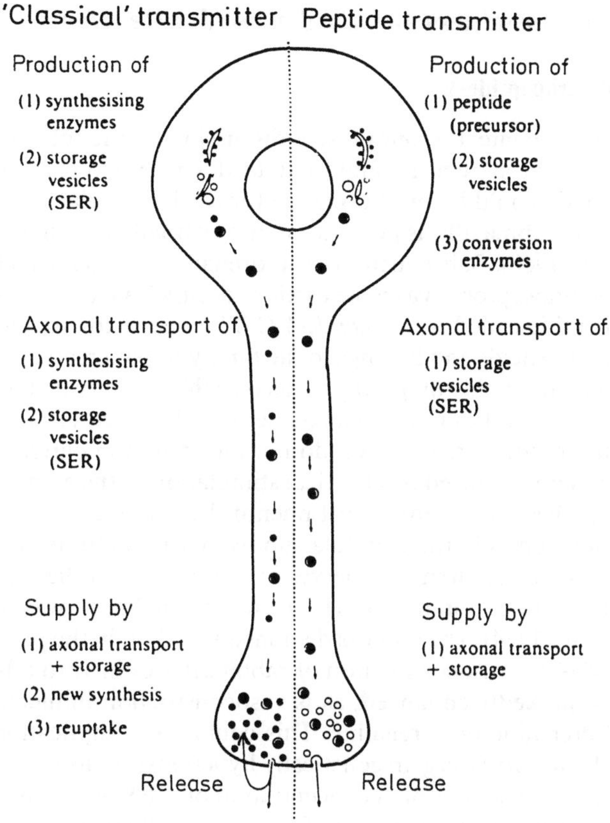

Fig. 4. Comparison of synthesis, transport, storage and release of a classical and peptide transmitter. *SER*, smooth endoplasmic reticulum (from Hökfelt et al. 1980, by permission of the publishers)

No re-uptake mechanism is likely, as it is known from the small molecules of noradrenaline or adrenaline in classical sympathetic neurones. Replenishment of peptide transmitter concentrations in neurones appears to be limited to axonal transport. This "slow mechanism" indicates another functional role compared with the classical transmitters, e.g. an intermittent release and a relatively long duration of action, perhaps thereby modulating the response to classical transmitters. Another feature of the peptides is activation of receptors at remarkably low concentrations, when compared with the relatively high concentrations of classical transmitters necessary for adrenoceptor activation.

The distribution of peptide containing neurones seems to be ubiquitous. In the central nervous system as well, gut hormones such as vasoactive intestinal peptide (VIP) and cholecystokinin (CCK) could be detected in coexistence with classical transmitters such as acetylcholine or dopamine (for details see Hökfelt et al. 1980; Grobecker 1983).

Cotransmitters and Cardiovascular Reactions

Neuropeptide-Y

In the context of our present discussion on the role of adrenoceptors in the cardiovascular system, I should like to describe two examples of coexistence situations which could be of importance for cardiovascular reactions. Arterioles of the glandula submaxillaris possess a dense sympathetic innervation (Grobecker and Malmfors 1968). Subsequent to noradrenaline release, which stimulates postsynaptic α-adrenoceptors, vasoconstriction occurs. As a cotransmitter in this situation, a peptide called *neuropeptide-Y* (NPY), seems to act. This peptide is composed of 36 amino acids and belongs to the family of pancreatic polypeptides. NPY was detected immunohistologically in nerves which innervate the same vessels in the submaxillary gland as noradrenergic nerves. However, NPY-containing nerves, in contrast to noradrenergic nerves, do not innervate the parenchyma of the gland. Vasoconstriction induced by electrical stimulation of the gland's peptide nerves could not be blocked by the antagonist phenoxybenzamine. The functional role played by peptide nerves in the glandula submaxillaris could be constriction of vessels independent of noradrenergic nerves or modulation of the release or action of the classical transmitter noradrenaline. The latter conclusion was recently supported by Ekblad et al. (1984). The authors demonstrated that, in the presence of small concentrations of NPY, vasoconstriction of rabbit arteries in vitro after electrical field stimulation is markedly enhanced, as is vasoconstriction induced by increasing doses of noradrenaline or adrenaline. This could have implications for the activity of sympathetic nerves, e.g. in genetically hypertensive rats or in young patients with essential hypertension. A high concentration of NPY was also reported in the superior cervical sympathetic ganglion of the cat (Lundberg et al. 1983). The same authors reported that intravenous injection of synthetic NPY in rats and cats caused a long-lasting elevation of blood pressure, which could not be blocked by α-adrenoceptor antagonists. This observation is in line with the conclusion drawn above concerning a possible implication of neuropeptides in hypertension.

A first report on immunohistochemically localized nerves containing NPY in the human heart was published by Gu et al. (1983). A dense innervation of NPY-immunoreactive fibres was found in association with nodal tissue and cardiac muscle fibres, as well as around the coronary vessels. Analysis of the peptide by high-performance liquid chromatography demonstrated that it was present in a single molecular form, closely similar or identical to that of the isolated bioactive peptide. One could speculate that NPY fibres are possibly involved in vasospasm of coronary arteries.

In addition, it is known that a denser innervation of arterioles with NPY containing neurones occurs, than that which is observed in venoles. Yet the action of NPY on cardiovascular parameters in humans remains to be elucidated.

Vasoactive Intestinal Polypeptide

Another peptide which occurs in a cotransmitter situation in neurones innervating vessels is vasoactive intestinal polypeptide (VIP). Its pharmacological action appears to be vasodilatation. After i.v. infusion of VIP in dogs, a long-lasting decrease in blood pressure was observed (Said and Mutt 1970). Immunohistochemical investigations by Larsson et al. (1976) showed a dense innervation of cerebral arteries by nerves containing VIP. In additional pharmacological investigations, the same authors reported a dose dependent vasodilatation in vitro in arteries contracted by pretreatment with serotonin. Even in concentrations of 3×10^{-10}M, VIP caused a vasodilatation which persisted for 15-20 min.

Physiological and Pharmacological Functions of Cotransmitters

In Table 1, several other known coexistence situations between classical transmitters and peptides are summarized (see also Hökfelt et al. 1984). According to these authors, peptides are mainly localized in vesicles with a mean diameter of 1000 Å, whereas catecholamines are preferentially stored in vesicles with a mean diameter of 500 Å. Depletion of the catecholamines by reserpine had no effect on, e.g. the storage of substance P (Hökfelt et al. 1984). Immunohistochemical investigations in combination with pharmacological experiments can provide us with some information about the functional or physiological role of the interaction between simultaneously or subsequently released cotransmitters.

In experiments on dogs, Hanbauer et al. (1982) demonstrated that enkephalins can inhibit the release of noradrenaline and adrenaline from the adrenal medulla. The interaction between enkephalins and the release of catecholamines probably

Table 1. Coexistence of Classical Transmitters and Peptides in Neurones (modified from Hökfelt et al. 1984)

Classical transmitter	Peptide	Tissue/region	Species
Dopamine	Enkephalin	Carotid body	Cat
	CCK	Ventral tegmental area	Rat, man
Noradrenaline	Somatostatin	Adrenal medulla	Man
	Enkephalin	Adrenal medulla	Several species
		Sympathetic ganglia	Rat
	Neurotensin	Adrenal medulla	Cat
	APP	Locus ceruleus	Rat
Adrenaline	Enkephalin	Adrenal medulla	Several species
	APP	Medulla oblongata	Rat
Serotonin	Substance P	Medulla oblongata	Rat
	TRH		
	Substance P and TRH		
GABA	Somatostatin	Thalamus	Cat

APP, avian pancreatic-like polypeptide; CCK, cholecystokinin-like peptide; TRH, thyroxin-releasing hormone; GABA, gamma-aminobutyric acid

Classical Transmitter
(Noradrenaline)
↓
Postsynaptic α, β-receptors ←—— **Presynaptic α, β-receptors**
↓
Regulatory component
(Guanine nucleotide)
↓
Adenylcyclase/Ca^{++}-channels

Cotransmitter
(Adrenaline, Peptide)
↓
Presynaptic α, β-receptors

Fig. 5. Role of cotransmitters in regulation of receptor entities (after Guidotti et al. 1983)

takes place on the level of the nicotinic receptors, which are stimulated by acetylcholine released from the splanchnic nerve.

A current hypothesis for possible interactions of two or more transmitters in a transmitter-cotransmitter entity is depicted in Fig. 5 (modified after Guidotti et al. 1983). Two populations of pharmacological receptors could be involved: firstly, peptides can act through classical adrenoceptors (α, β), e.g. by modifying the operation of the regulator protein or their subpopulations (α_1, α_2, β_1, β_2) or secondly, they act on specific receptors, reserved for the action of peptides, thereby modulating the release of a classical transmitter beyond the adrenergic receptor level.

In summary, results of experiments, mainly from laboratories in Sweden and the United States, concerning the function of cotransmitters and classical transmitters allow the conclusion that a peptide cotransmitter stored and released together with classical transmitters will generally modify the action of a classical transmitter. In order to obtain more information about these important pharmacological cardiovascular actions of peptide-cotransmitters, it is necessary to develop specific antagonists against the effect of peptides (cf. Jensen et al. 1984), following the line of the classical concept of agonist-antagonist interactions in the field of adrenoceptors.

References

Brown MJ (1984) The role of adrenaline in essential hypertension in man. Iuphar 9th International congress of pharmacology, London, Abstract L12

Burnstock G, Sneddon P (1985) Evidence for ATP and noradrenaline as co-transmitters in sympathetic nerves. Clin Sci 68 [Suppl 10]: 89s-92s

Dominiak P, Grobecker H (1982) Elevated plasma catecholamines in young hypertensive and hyperkinetic patients: effect of pindolol. Br J Clin Pharmacol 13: 381S-390S

Ekblad E, Edvinsson L, Wahlestedt C, Uddman R, Hakanson R, Sundler F (1984) Neuropeptide-Y co-exists and co-operates with noradrenaline in perivascular nerve fibers. Regul Peptides 8: 225-235

Grobecker H (1983) Transmitter-peptide coexistence in the central nervous system. Eur Neurol 22 [Suppl 1]: 38-46

Grobecker H, Malmfors T (1968) Fluorescenzmikroskopische Untersuchungen über die Wirkung des Prenylamins auf noradrenergische Nerven. Naunyn-Schmiedebergs Arch Pharmakol Exp Pathol 261: 59-74

Gu J, Adrian TE, Tatemoto K, Polak JM, Allen JM, Bloom SR (1983) Neuropeptide tyrosine (NPY) - a major cardiac neuropeptide. Lancet 1: 1008-1010

Guidotti A, Saiani L, Wise BC, Costa E (1983) Co-transmitters: pharmacological implications. J Neurotrans 18: 213-225

Hanbauer J, Kelly GD, Saiani L, Yang HYT (1982) Met-enkephalin like peptides of the adrenal medulla: release by nerve stimulation and functional implications. Peptides 3: 469-473

Hökfelt T, Johansson O, Ljungdahl R, Lundberg JM, Schultzberg M (1980) Peptidergic neurones. Nature 284 (5756): 515-521

Hökfelt T, Johansson O, Goldstein M (1984) Chemical anatomy of the brain. Science 225: 1326-1334

Hughes J, Smith TW, Kosterlitz HW, Forthergill LA, Morgan BA, Morris HR (1975) Identification of two related pentapeptides from the brain with potent opiate agonist activity. Nature 258: 577-579

Jensen RR, Jones SW, Folkers K, Gardner JD (1984) A synthetic peptide that is a bombesin receptor antagonist. Nature 309 (5963): 61-63

Larsson LJ, Childers SR, Snyder SH (1979) Met- and Leu-enkephalin immunoreactivity in separate neurones. Nature 282: 407-410

Larsson LJ, Edvinsson L, Fahrenkrug J, Hakanson R, Owman C, Schaffalitzky de Muckadell O, Sundler F (1976) Immunohistological localization of a vasodilatory polypeptide (VIP) in cerebrovascular nerves. Brain Res 113: 400-404

Lundberg JM, Hökfelt T, Tatemoto K, Terenius L (1983) Interaction of catecholamines and peptides in control of peripheral circulation. 5th CA-Symposion, Göteborg 1983. Prog Neuropsychopharmacol Biol Psychiatry 42 [Suppl]: 22

Rand MJ, Majewski H, Tung LH (1983) Activation of prejunctional β-adrenoceptors by adrenaline acting as a co-transmitter - a possible cause of hypertension. Drugs 25 [Suppl 2]: 64-68

Said SI, Mutt V (1970) Potent peripheral and splanchnic vasodilator peptide from normal gut. Nature 225: 863-864

Schümann HJ (1958) Über den Noradrenalin- und ATP-Gehalt sympathetischer Nerven. Naunyn-Schmiedebergs Arch Pharmacol 233: 296-300

II. Adrenoceptors of the Cardiovascular Musculature

Adrenoceptors in the Myocardium: Mechanical and Biochemical Events Resulting from Their Stimulation*

H. Scholz

Abteilung Allgemeine Pharmakologie, Universitäts-Krankenhaus Eppendorf, Martinistraße 52, 2000 Hamburg 20, Federal Republic of Germany

Adrenaline and noradrenaline increase the force of contraction of the heart (positive inotropic effect) and the heart rate (positive chronotropic effect). They also lead to an increase in the rate of relaxation and, hence, to an abbreviation of the contraction (relaxant effect). The physiological relevance of the relaxant effects of the sympathomimetic agents has been fully recognized only recently; it permits adequate ventricular filling in the face of the increased heart rate.

It is generally accepted that all of the effects mentioned above are mainly mediated by β-adrenoceptors. However, more recent evidence suggests that α-adrenoceptors are also present in the myocardium and that stimulation of these sites mainly exerts an increase in force of contraction. The first papers on α-adrenoceptor-mediated positive inotropic effects were published by Wenzel and Su (1966), Govier (1967) and Benfey and Varma (1967).

This short review is concerned with the mechanisms of the positive inotropic effects produced by stimulation of β- and α-adrenoceptors. The adrenoceptors involved are postsynaptic and are mainly of the β_1- and α_1-type respectively. More detailed information on the mechanisms of the positive inotropic effects mediated by myocardial β- or α-adrenoceptors may be found in a variety of recent reviews to which the reader is referred (Tsien 1977; Wollenberger and Will 1978; Drummond and Severson 1979, Katz 1979; Osnes et al. 1980; Benfey 1980, 1982; Scholz 1980, 1984; Schümann 1980; Endoh 1982; Reuter 1983; Brückner et al. 1985).

Mechanism of the β-Adrenergic Positive Inotropic Effect

The mechanism of the positive inotropic action of β-sympathomimetic agents is still hypothetical in some details. However, there is general agreement that these drugs ultimately lead to an increase in intracellular free Ca^{++} to interact with the contractile proteins (more exactly: with the Ca^{++} acceptor troponin C), that they increase the cAMP content of the heart and that the actions on both the Ca^{++} and the cyclic adenosine monophosphate (cAMP) system are causally related to each other. The present view on the mechanism of action of β-sympathomimetic agents is illustrated by the unifying scheme shown in Fig. 1.

The main effect of β-adrenergic agents is to enhance the entry of Ca^{++} into the myocardial cell during the excitation process. This has been shown by tracer studies

* Research from the author's laboratory was supported by the *Deutsche Forschungsgemeinschaft*

New Aspects of the Role of Adrenoceptors in the Cardiovascular System/Ed. by Grobecker et al.

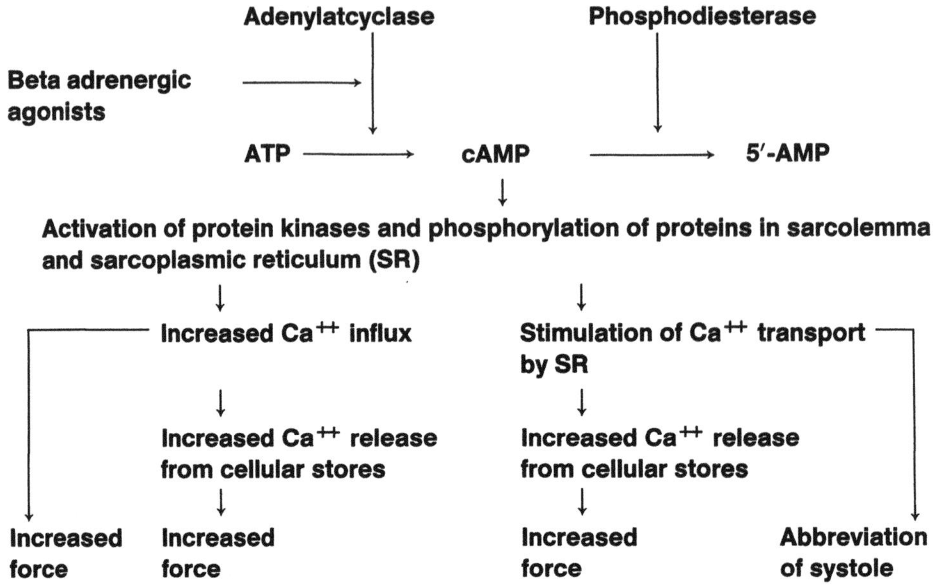

Fig. 1. Summary of the reactions through which β-adrenergic agents may lead to an increase in force of contraction (positive inotropic effect) and to a decrease in the duration of the contraction (relaxant effect) in the mammalian heart

with $^{45}Ca^{++}$ and by electrophysiological experiments where an increase in slow inward current has been directly demonstrated with the voltage clamp method or, less directly, by measuring the rate of rise of Ca^{++}-dependent slow action potentials. It has also been shown that the β-adrenergic effects on slow Ca^{++} inward current or Ca^{++}-dependent action potentials and on force of contraction are similarly related to time and concentration. It is still not clear how the increase in slow Ca^{++} inward current leads to the increase in force of contraction. It seems unlikely that it directly increases the Ca^{++} concentration at the contractile proteins to a major degree. Instead, the increase in slow Ca^{++} inward current predominantly leads to an increased Ca^{++} release from intracellular stores (presumably the sarcoplasmic reticulum), either because it serves as a greater trigger for a Ca^{++}-dependent Ca^{++} release or because it increases the filling of these stores with Ca^{++} that can be released during subsequent beats.

In addition to the increase in slow Ca^{++} inward current, β-adrenergic agonists lead to an increase in Ca^{++} uptake into the sarcoplasmic reticulum, which also increases the amount of releasable Ca^{++} within these stores. This increase in Ca^{++} uptake by the sarcoplasmic reticulum not only contributes to the positive inotropic properties, but also explains the relaxant effects of the β-adrenergic agonists. However, there is some evidence that the latter might, in part, also be due to a decrease in the Ca^{++} sensitivity of the contractile proteins (cf. Katz 1979; Osnes et al. 1980).

A question which arises is which biochemical reactions may mediate the abovementioned β-adrenergic effects on the Ca^{++} movements during the myocardial contraction-relaxation cycle.

It is generally accepted that β-adrenergic agents increase the myocardial cAMP content and that this cAMP-increasing action precedes the positive inotropic effect. Moreover, the positive inotropic effect of β-adrenergic agents is increased by phosphodiesterase inhibitors (e.g. theophylline) and mimicked by cAMP derivatives. All of these findings support the view that the increase in cAMP content and force of contraction are causally related to each other. cAMP causes an activation of protein kinases and, as a result, the phosphorylation of several proteins. This changes the functional properties of the proteins, for example their ability to bind Ca^{++} ions, and may thus explain the β-adrenergic effects on the Ca^{++} movements in the sarcoplasmic reticulum and possibly also in the sarcolemma.

The mechanism of the cAMP-dependent activation of protein kinases has also been elucidated. The enzyme consists of two subunits: a regulatory subunit which binds cAMP and a catalytic subunit. In the absence of cAMP, both subunits form an enzymatically inactive complex. The binding of cAMP by the regulatory subunit prevents the inhibitory action of the catalytic subunit.

That the cAMP-dependent phosphorylation of functional proteins is related to myocardial Ca^{++} movements has first been detected in isolated sarcoplasmic reticulum preparations. The increase in Ca^{++} uptake into these structures results from a cAMP-dependent phosphorylation of phospholamban. The β-adrenergic effect on the slow Ca^{++} inward current possibly also results from a cAMP-dependent phosphorylation of proteins in the sarcolemma. Finally, the decrease in the Ca^{++} sensitivity of the contractile proteins is probably also brought about by a cAMP-dependent protein phosphorylation, namely a phosphorylation of troponin I.

In summary, the positive inotropic effect of β-adrenergic agents is mainly due to an increase in slow Ca^{++} inward current and in Ca^{++} uptake into the sarcoplasmic reticulum. These effects, in turn, are presumably due to a cAMP-dependent phosphorylation of a variety of functional proteins. Hence, the β-adrenergic effects on myocardial Ca^{++} movements on the one hand and on the cAMP system on the other are probably causally related in a common pathway, where the β-adrenergic drug represents the first messenger and cAMP and Ca^{++} are the second and third messengers respectively.

The β-adrenergic effect of increasing the slow Ca^{++} inward current has originally been attributed to an increase in the number of functional Ca^{++} channels (Reuter and Scholz 1977). More recently, however, using the patch clamp method to record current flow through single channels, it has become evident that β-adrenergic agents increase the probability of Ca^{++} channels to open during depolarization. Figure 2, modified from a recent review by Siegelbaum and Tsien (1983), illustrates schematically that an increase in current flow through a population of channels may be brought about in three ways. It may be due (a) to an increase in the total number of functional channels, (b) to an increase in current flowing through an open individual channel and (c) to an increase in the probability that an individual channel is in the open state. β-Adrenergic agents probably increase the slow Ca^{++} inward current in the latter way (Reuter et al. 1982; Reuter 1983; Siegelbaum and Tsien 1983; Hess et al. 1984).

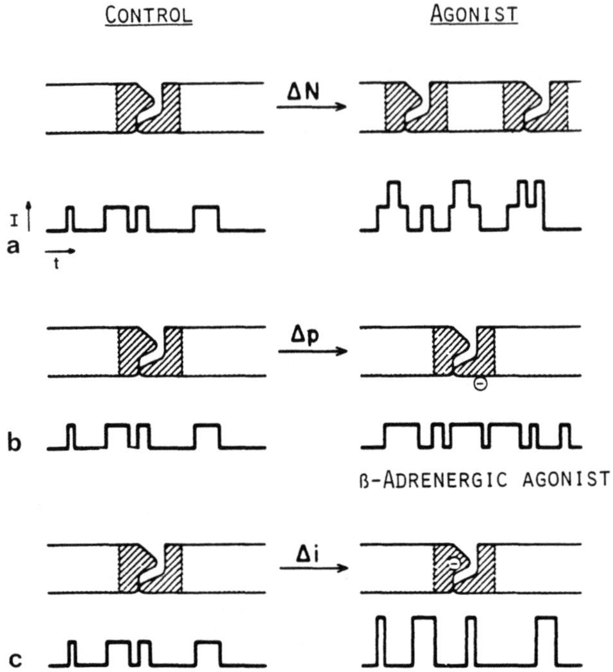

Fig. 2a–c. Schematic illustration of the possibilities through which a current through a population of channels may be increased. *β*-Adrenergic agents probably affect the opening behaviour of single Ca^{++} channels. They increase the probability that Ca^{++} channels are in the open state. This leads to an increase in slow Ca^{++} inward current. Modified from Siegelbaum and Tsien (1983).
The overall current *I* through a population of channels is given by $N \cdot p \cdot i$: *N*, total number of functional channels; *p*, probability that an individual channel is open; *i*, current through an open individual channel

Mechanism of the *α*-Adrenergic Positive Inotropic Effect

There is no doubt that the positive inotropic response to adrenergic agents in the heart is mediated predominantly by *β*-adrenoceptors. However, it is now generally accepted that *α*-adrenoceptors also exist in the myocardium and that an increase in force of contraction may be produced by stimulation of these sites. *α*-Adrenoceptors producing positive inotropic effects have been found in most species, including man. The positive inotropic effect of *α*-adrenergic agents is qualitatively different from that of *β*-adrenergic drugs. The *α*-adrenergic response develops relatively slowly and is not accompanied by a shortening but, instead, by a prolongation of the contraction. Thus, *α*-adrenergic agents do not produce relaxant effects. Moreover, the *α*-adrenergic positive inotropic effect is dependent on the heart rate. It is nearly absent at stimulation frequencies below 0.1 Hz and higher than 4 Hz and is most evident at the relatively low frequency of about 1 Hz. In addition, the *α*-adrenergic effect is more pronounced in hypothyroidism than under normal conditions. Another difference between *α*- and *β*-adrenergic positive inotropic effects is that the

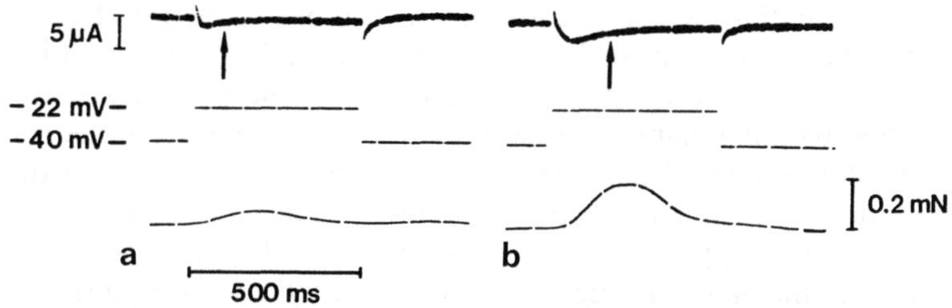

Fig. 3 a, b. Effect of phenylephrine in the presence of propranolol on the slow Ca^{++} inward current. Voltage clamp experiment in a bovine electrically driven right-ventricular trabecula. *Uppermost trace,* membrane current; downward deflection denotes inward current. The arrows denote the time constant of the inactivation of the slow inward current. *Middle trace,* membrane potential; clamp step from a holding potential of -40 mV to -22 mV for 500 ms. *Lowermost trace,* force of contraction. Frequency of stimulation 0.3 Hz. Propranolol 1 μmol l^{-1} was present throughout. *a,* control; *b,* phenylephrine 10 μmol l^{-1}, incubation time 10 min. Modified from Brückner and Scholz (1984)

latter, but not the former, can be impaired by cholinergic agents or adenosine. Carbachol or adenosine, for instance, are capable of decreasing the β-adrenoceptor-mediated positive inotropic effect of isoprenaline; however, the positive inotropic effect of phenylephrine or methoxamine mediated by α-adrenoceptors is not affected under these conditions (Endoh and Motomura 1979; Endoh and Yamashita 1980).

The mechanism of the α-adrenergic positive inotropic response is unknown. It is generally accepted, however, that there is no increase in cAMP levels, quite in accordance with the observation that there is no relaxant effect. cGMP levels and $(Na^+ + K^+)$-adenosine triphosphatase (ATPase) activity also remain unchanged.

It is generally accepted that an increase in the force of myocardial contraction may be ultimately due to two basic effects: (a) an increase in intracellular free Ca^{++} to interact with the contractile proteins and (b) an increased sensitivity of the myofilaments for Ca^{++}. Therefore, we have investigated whether or not α-adrenergic agents lead to an increase in slow Ca^{++} inward current as do β-sympathomimetic drugs. The effect of phenylephrine on Ca^{++}-dependent slow action potentials has been investigated where the rate of depolarization can be taken as an indirect measure of the size of the slow Ca^{++} inward current. Direct measurements of the slow Ca^{++} inward current with the voltage clamp method were also performed. The results of these studies have recently been published in detail (Brückner and Scholz 1984). In brief, phenylephrine in the presence of propranolol led to an increase in the maximal rate of depolarization of slow action potentials. All effects of phenylephrine were abolished by the α-adrenoceptor blocking agent phentolamine. In the voltage clamp experiment (Fig. 3), phenylephrine increased the magnitude of the slow Ca^{++} inward current. In addition, the decay of the slow Ca^{++} inward current was decelerated so that the slow Ca^{++} inward current was increased, not only with respect to its magnitude, but also in its duration. Finally, we compared the effects of phenylephrine with those of the β-adrenergic agent isoprenaline. At concentrations producing similar positive inotropic effects, the increase in slow Ca^{++} inward current was much less pronounced than that produced by isoprenaline (Brückner and Scholz 1984).

These findings are in accordance with those of Miura et al. (1978), who have found that phenylephrine in the presence of the β-adrenoceptor blocking agent bufetolol elicited slow action potentials in rabbit papillary muscles which were blocked by phentolamine. However, they are in contrast to the results of Ledda et al. (1980) and Sanchez-Chapula (1981). These authors found that the effects of phenylephrine on Ca^{++}-dependent slow action potentials in guinea-pig papillary muscles were suppressed by β-adrenoceptor blocking agents and were hence apparently not mediated through α-, but through β-adrenoceptors. These differences, however, can probably be related to species differences. According to functional studies by Shibata et al. (1980), α-adrenoceptors are only of minor importance or are but poorly developed in guinea-pig ventricular tissues.

In summary, it is quite conceivable that an increase in slow Ca^{++} inward current at least contributes to the positive inotropic effect of α-sympathomimetic agents. However, since the α-adrenergic increase in slow Ca^{++} inward current is relatively small, as compared with that produced by β-adrenergic agents, other (still unknown) mechanisms are probably also involved. Endoh and Blinks (1984), using the bioluminescent protein aequorin, have recently shown that phenylephrine increases the Ca^{++} sensitivity of contractile proteins. This finding would fit very well into the above-mentioned hypothesis.

As in the case of the β-adrenergic positive inotropic effect, a question that arises is which biochemical reactions or events are responsible for the positive inotropic effect brought about by stimulation of α-adrenoceptors. Figure 4 illustrates possible mechanisms of the α-adrenergic positive inotropic action. The above-mentioned increase in slow Ca^{++} inward current *(1)* is apparently independent of an increase in cAMP. The increase in slow Ca^{++} inward current presumably exerts an increased release of Ca^{++} from intracellular stores *(2)*. Ca^{++} released from intracellular stores in turn possibly modulates the slow Ca^{++} inward current *(6)*. If this were true, the increase in slow Ca^{++}-inward current produced by α-adrenergic agents would not completely be due to direct, but also to indirect mechanisms. This possibility was first discussed by Kass et al. (1978), Kass and Tsien (1982) and Marban and Tsien (1982) in the context of their studies on the mechanism of the positive inotropic effects of cardiac glycosides. Step 3 in Figure 4 denotes the above-mentioned increase in the Ca^{++} sensitivity of the contractile proteins. However, still other mechanisms must be discussed. Michell (1975, 1979) proposed that all agents which cAMP-independently increase the Ca^{++} concentration within the cell also produce an increase in phosphatidylinositol turnover. In this scheme, the increased phosphatidylinositol turnover is possibly not a result but, instead, the cause of the increase in the Ca^{++} concentration in the cytosol. It has been shown in a variety of tissues (e.g. smooth muscle, platelets, salivary glands, liver and pancreas) that the stimulation of different receptors, for instance the α-adrenoceptor, may lead to an increase in Ca^{++} concentration in the cytosol as a result of an increased breakdown of membrane-bound phosphoinositides (for references, see Fain and García-Saínz 1980; Nishizuka 1983; Michell 1983; Berridge 1984; Berridge and Irvine 1984; Farese 1984). Here, phosphatidylinositol 4,5-bisphosphate is hydrolized to a greater amount into the breakdown products inositol trisphosphate and diacylglycerol, which then possibly function as "second messengers" within the cell (step 4 in Figure 4). Inositol trisphosphate seems to be capable of mobilizing Ca^{++} from the sarcoplasmic reticulum

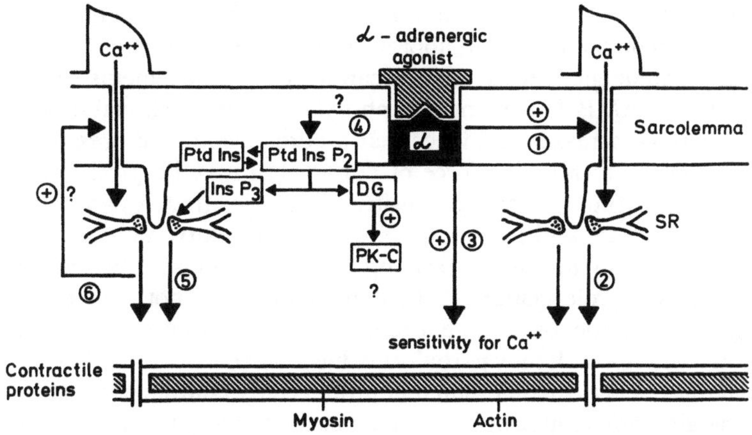

Fig. 4. Schematic illustration of possible mechanisms underlying the α-adrenergic positive inotropic effect in the mammalian heart. *1,* Stimulation of α-adrenoceptors produces a cAMP-independent increase in slow Ca^{++} inward current. *2,* The increase in slow Ca^{++} inward current leads to an increase in Ca^{++} release from intracellular stores, presumably the sarcoplasmatic reticulum *(SR). 3,* Additional stimulation of α-adrenoceptors may lead to increased Ca^{++} sensitivity of the contractile proteins. *4,* It seems possible that α-adrenoceptors and phosphatidylinositol turnover are related to each other also in the heart. Stimulation of α-adrenoceptors may lead to an increased breakdown of phosphatidylinositol 4,5-bisphosphate. The reaction products are inositol trisphosphate and diacylglycerol. *5,* Inositoltrisphosphate possibly releases Ca^{++} from the SR. *6,* Ca^{++} released from the SR is presumably involved in the regulation of the slow Ca^{++} inward current. +, stimulation; *Ptd Ins,* phosphatidylinositol; *Ptd Ins* P_2, phosphatidylinositol 4,5-bisphosphate; *Ins* P_3, inositol trisphosphate; *SR,* sarcoplasmic reticulum; *DG,* diacylglycerol; *PK-C,* protein kinase C. Modified from Brückner et al. (1985)

(step 5 in Fig. 4). Diacylglycerol obviously activates the Ca^{++}-dependent protein kinase C, the functional importance of which in the heart, however, remains to be elucidated.

Recent experiments have provided evidence that the above-mentioned phosphatidylinositol pathway may also be operative as a basis for the α-adrenergic positive inotropic action in the heart. Uchida et al. (1982) and Quist and Sanchez (1983) reported that stimulation of α-adrenoceptors in rat and canine myocardial tissues produced an increased rate of ^{32}P uptake into phosphatidylinositol and phosphatidic acid. However, it remains to be elucidated whether the increased phosphatidylinositol turnover in the heart is only an event accompanying α-adrenoceptor stimulation or whether it is in fact causally related to the α-adrenergic positive inotropic effect.

Summary

There is no doubt that the positive inotropic effect of adrenergic agents in the mammalian heart is predominantly mediated by β-adrenoceptors. The β-adrenergic positive inotropic action is mainly due to an increase in slow Ca^{++} inward current during the action potential and to an increased uptake of Ca^{++} into the sarcoplasmic reticulum. The latter action also explains that the β-adrenergic positive inotropic effect is accompanied by an abbreviation of the contraction (relaxant effect). All of the β-adrenergic effects on myocardial Ca^{++} movements are probably brought about by cAMP-dependent phosphorylations of functional proteins.

There is increasing evidence that α-adrenoceptors also exist in the myocardium and that an increase in force of contraction may be produced by stimulation of these sites. The α-adrenergic positive inotropic effect is particularly pronounced at low heart rates and in hypothyroidism. It develops more slowly than the β-adrenergic positive inotropic effect and is not accompanied by an abbreviation but, instead, by a prolongation of the contraction. It is not antagonized by cholinergic agents or by adenosine. The mechanisms of the α-adrenergic positive inotropic action is unknown. It may partially be due to an increase in slow Ca^{++} inward current, but this effect is smaller than that produced by β-adrenergic compounds. The α-adrenergic positive inotropic effect is not related to an increase in myocardial cAMP levels. An increase in the Ca^{++} sensitivity of the contractile proteins may also contribute to the positive inotropic effect of α-adrenergic agents. Another unknown issue is whether or not the α-adrenergic positive inotropic action is related to an increased turnover of phosphatidylinositol, which in other tissues has been found to release Ca^{++} from intracellular stores.

References

Benfey BG (1980) Cardiac α-adrenoceptors. Can J Physiol Pharmacol 58: 1145-1157

Benfey BG (1982) Function of myocardial alpha adrenoceptors. In: Riemersma RA, Oliver MF (eds) Catecholamines in the non-ischaemic and ischaemic myocardium. Elsevier, Amsterdam, pp 41-57

Benfey BG, Varma DR (1967) Interactions of sympathomimetic drugs, propranolol and phentolamine, on atrial refractory period and contractility. Br J Pharmacol 30: 603-611

Berridge MJ (1984) Inositol trisphosphate and diacylglycerol as second messengers. Biochem J 220: 345-360

Berridge MJ, Irvine RF (1984) Inositol trisphosphate, a novel second messenger in cellular signal transduction. Nature 312: 315-321

Brückner R, Mügge A, Scholz H (1985) Existence and functional role of $alpha_1$-adrenoceptors in the mammalian heart. J Mol Cell Cardiol 17: 639-645

Brückner R, Scholz H (1984) Effects of α-adrenoceptor stimulation with phenylephrine in the presence of propranolol on force of contraction, slow inward current and cyclic AMP content in the bovine heart. Br J Pharmacol 82: 223-232

Drummond GI, Severson DL (1979) Cyclic nucleotides and cardiac function. Circ Res 44: 145-153

Endoh M (1982) Adrenoceptors and the myocardial inotropic response: do alpha and beta receptor sites functionally coexist? In: Kalsner S (ed) Trends in autonomic pharmacology, vol 2. Urban and Schwarzenberg, Baltimore, pp 303-322

Endoh M, Blinks JR (1984) Regulation of the intracellular Ca^{++} transient and Ca^{++}-sensitivity of myofibrils via α- and β-adrenoceptors in the rabbit papillary muscle. Cell Calcium 5: 301

Endoh M, Motomura S (1979) Differentiation by cholinergic stimulation of positive inotropic actions mediated via α- and β-adrenoceptors in the rabbit heart. Life Sci 25: 759-768

Endoh M, Yamashita S (1980) Adenosine antagonizes the positive inotropic action mediated via β-, but not α-adrenoceptors in the rabbit papillary muscle. Eur J Pharmacol 65: 445-448

Fain JN, García-Sáinz JA (1980) Role of phosphatidylinositol turnover in $alpha_1$ and of adenylate cyclase inhibition in $alpha_2$ effects of catecholamines. Life Sci 26: 1183-1194

Farese RV (1984) Phospholipids as intermediates in hormone action. Mol Cell Endocrinol 35: 1-14

Govier WC (1967) A positive inotropic effect of phenylephrine mediated through alpha adrenergic receptors. Life Sci 6: 1361-1365

Hess P, Lansman JB, Tsien RW (1984) Different modes of Ca channel gating behaviour favoured by dihydropyridine Ca agonists and antagonists. Nature 311: 538-544

Kass RS, Lederer WJ, Tsien RW, Weingart R (1978) Role of calcium ions in transient inward currents and aftercontractions induced by strophanthidin in cardiac Purkinje fibres. J Physiol (Lond) 281: 187-208

Kass RS, Tsien RW (1982) Fluctuations in membrane current driven by intracellular calcium in cardiac Purkinje fibers. Biophys J 38: 259-269

Katz AM (1979) Role of the contractile proteins and sarcoplasmic reticulum in the response of the heart to catecholamines: an historical review. Adv Cyclic Nucleotide Res 11: 303-343

Ledda F, Mantelli L, Mugelli A (1980) α-Sympathomimetic amines and calcium-mediated action potentials in guinea-pig ventricular muscle. Br J Pharmacol 69: 565-571

Marban E, Tsien RW (1982) Enhancement of calcium current during digitalis inotropy in mammalian heart: positive feed-back regulation by intracellular calcium? J Physiol (Lond) 329: 589-614

Michell RH (1975) Inositol phospholipids and cell surface receptor function. Biochim Biophys Acta 415: 81-147

Michell RH (1979) Inositol phospholipids in membrane function. Trends Biochem Sci 4: 128-131

Michell RH (1983) Polyphosphoinositide breakdown as the initiating reaction in receptor-stimulated inositol phospholipid metabolism. Life Sci 32: 2083-2085

Miura Y, Inui J, Imamura H (1978) Alpha-adrenoceptor-mediated restoration of calcium-dependent potential in the partially depolarized rabbit papillary muscle. Naunyn-Schmiedebergs Arch Pharmacol 301: 201-205

Nishizuka Y (1983) Phospholipid degradation and signal translation for protein phosphorylation. Trends Biochem Sci 8: 13-16

Osnes JB, Skomedal T, Øye I (1980) On the role of cyclic nucleotides in the heart muscle contraction and relaxation. Prog Pharmacol 4: 47-62

Quist E, Sanchez M (1983) Alpha adrenergic drugs induce a phospholipid effect in canine heart. Proc West Pharmacol Soc 26: 333-335

Reuter H (1983) Calcium channel modulation by neurotransmitters, enzymes and drugs. Nature 301: 569-574

Reuter H, Scholz H (1977) The regulation of the calcium conductance of cardiac muscle by adrenaline. J Physiol (Lond) 264: 49-62

Reuter H, Stevens CF, Tsien RW, Yellen G (1982) Properties of single calcium channels in cardiac cell culture. Nature 297: 501-504

Sanchez-Chapula J (1981) Multiple effects of putative α-adrenoceptor agonists on the electrical and mechanical activity of guinea-pig papillary muscle. Naunyn-Schmiedebergs Arch Pharmacol 316: 108-111

Scholz H (1980) Effects of beta- and alpha-adrenoceptor activators and adrenergic transmitter releasing agents on the mechanical activity of the heart. In: Szekeres L (ed) Adrenergic activators and inhibitors, part 1. Springer, Berlin Heidelberg New York, pp 651-733 (Handbook of experimental pharmacology, vol 54/I)

Scholz H (1984) Inotropic drugs and their mechanisms of action. J Am Coll Cardiol 4: 389-397

Schümann HJ (1980) Are there α-adrenoceptors in the mammalian heart? Trends Pharmacol Sci 1: 195-197

Shibata S, Seriguchi DG, Iwadare S, Ishida Y, Shibata T (1980) The regional and species differences on the activation of myocardial alpha-adrenoceptors by phenylephrine and methoxamine. Gen Pharmacol 11: 173-180

Siegelbaum SA, Tsien RW (1983) Modulation of gated ion channels as a mode of transmitter action. Trends Neurosci 6: 307-313

Tsien RW (1977) Cyclic AMP and contractile activity in heart. Adv Cyclic Nucleotide Res 8: 363-420

Uchida T, Bhatnagar GM, Lakatta EG, Filburn CR (1982) Alpha-adrenergic stimulation of $^{32}PO_4$ labelling of phosphatidylinositol (PI) and phosphatidic acid (PA) in cultured rat heart cells. Fed Proc 41: 1523

Wenzel DG, Su JL (1966) Interactions between sympathomimetic amines and blocking agents on the rat ventricle strip. Arch Int Pharmacodyn Ther 160: 379-389

Wollenberger A, Will H (1978) Protein kinase-catalyzed membrane phosphorylation and its possible relationship to the role of calcium in the adrenergic regulation of cardiac contraction. Life Sci 22: 1159-1178

Regulation of Myocardial Contractility Via Adrenoceptors: Differential Mechanisms of α- and β-Adrenoceptor-Mediated Actions*

M. Endoh

Department of Pharmacology, Yamagata University School of Medicine, Nishinomae, Zao-iida, 990-23 Yamagata, Japan

Introduction

The force of myocardial contraction is regulated primarily by catecholamines released from sympathetic nerve endings and adrenal glands through nerve excitation which adjust the cardiac function to the momentary physical requirement. Molecules of the released catecholamines bind to adrenoceptors located on the outer surface of the myocardial cell membrane and initiate a series of biochemical processes, which result in the characteristic changes in mechanical performance. It is generally agreed that the adrenoceptor predominantly involved in the regulation of myocardial contractility is of the β-type. The subcellular biochemical processes that follow the activation of β-adrenoceptors induced by the binding of sympathomimetic amines have been well documented in the past two decades. It is beyond the scope of this paper to review the β-adrenoceptor-mediated mechanism in detail. It will be described only as far as is necessary to permit comparison with the rather different subcellular processes that appear to result from myocardial α-adrenoceptor stimulation.

It has been established that the stimulation of β-adrenoceptors by sympathomimetic amines leads to an accumulation of adenosine 3',5'-cyclic monophosphate (cyclic AMP) in the myocardial cells through modulation of the stimulatory guanine nucleotide regulatory protein (N_s). This results in the activation of the catalytic subunit of membrane-bound adenylate cyclase (Smigel et al. 1984; Lefkowitz et al. 1984; Spiegel et al. 1985). Cyclic AMP accumulated intracellularly in turn promotes the phosphorylation of diverse functional proteins of various structures of myocardial cells, i. e. sarcolemma, sarcoplasmic recticulum (phospholamban) and thin filaments (troponin I). As a result, Ca^{++} influx via the sarcolemma increases, the rate of Ca^{++} uptake into the sarcoplasmic reticulum increases and the Ca^{++} sensitivity of contractile apparatus (troponin C) decreases. The net effect of these changes is an increase in strength of myocardial contraction, associated with acceleration of relaxation and abbreviation of contraction (for reviews, see Tsien 1977; Solaro 1982; Katz 1983; Demaille et al. 1983; Winegrad 1984).

On the other hand, since the late 1960s it has been clearly shown that in certain types of mammalian and amphibian myocardium, the positive inotropic actions of sympathomimetic amines can be mediated by myocardial α-adrenoceptors in addition to the predominant β-adrenoceptors (for reviews, see Benfey 1980; Scholz

* Supported in part by USPHS Grant HL 12186

New Aspects of the Role of Adrenoceptors in the Cardiovascular System/Ed. by Grobecker et al.

1980; Schümann 1980; Endoh 1982). Although the subcellular mechanism underlying the positive inotropic action mediated via α-adrenoceptors is much less well understood than the β-adrenoceptor-mediated intracellular process, I will try in this paper to delineate the mechanisms that allow the influence of myocardial α-adrenoceptor stimulation to be expressed by contrasting the effects of α- and β-adrenoceptor stimulation on biochemical, electrophysiological and mechanical responses.

Characteristics of Myocardial α-Adrenoceptors

Since the classification of binding sites of myocardial β-adrenoceptors is considered in detail elsewhere (see O. Brodde, this volume), I will focus on the characteristics of the class of α-adrenoceptor binding sites involved in the regulation of myocardial contractility. The direct identification of myocardial α-adrenoceptors by radioligand binding studies confirmed and extended earlier evidence for the functional existence of α-adrenoceptors. Firstly, it was shown that a potent α-adrenoceptor antagonist, [^{3}H]dihydroergocryptine, bound specifically and with high affinity to a particulate membrane fraction derived from rat (Williams and Lefkowitz 1978; Guicheney et al. 1978) and rabbit (Schümann and Brodde 1979) myocardium. The binding site had the characteristics expected of α-adrenoceptors with respect to the stereospecific displacement of the tritiated ligand by α-adrenoceptor agonists and antagonists. Soon thereafter, it was further shown that a specific α_1-adrenoceptor antagonist, [^{3}H]prazosin, but not an α_2-antagonist, [^{3}H]yohimbine bound with high specificity to the particulate membrane fractions of guinea pig and rat hearts (Karliner et al. 1979; Mukherjee et al. 1983) and to intact cells isolated from adult rat hearts (Skomedal et al. 1984). Mukherjee et al. (1983) examined the number of myocardial α_1-adrenoceptor binding sites in various mammalian species and found markedly fewer α_1-adrenoceptors and more β-adrenoceptor binding sites (B_{max}) in dog than in rabbit or rat myocardium. These findings are consistent with the previous functional observations in the dog myocardium that the positive inotropic effects of sympathomimetic amines are mostly mediated by β-adrenoceptors (Endoh et al. 1978; Yamashita and Endoh 1981). In the guinea pig, in which the α-mediated positive inotropic action is less pronounced than in the rat or rabbit (Shibata et al. 1980), the number of α_1-adrenoceptor binding sites in the myocardial cell membrane (58 fmol/mg protein, Karliner et al. 1979) is similar to the level in the dog myocardial cell membrane (55 fmol/mg protein; Mukherjee et al. 1983). These observations imply that the functional significance of α-adrenoceptors in mediating the positive inotropic action of sympathomimetic amines in different mammalian species is dependent on the number of α_1-adrenoceptor binding sites in the individual species. On the other hand, the characteristics of myocardial α-adrenoceptors mediating the positive inotropic action are different from the prototype of α_1-adrenoceptors (e.g. in vascular smooth muscle). Certain potent α_1-agonists such as oxymetazoline and naphazoline are incapable or only slightly capable of increasing the strength of myocardial contraction, but inhibit the α-mediated positive inotropic action in a competitive manner (Fig. 1). This implies that the subclass of the *binding site* of myocardial α-adrenoceptors may be α_1-subtype, but that the coupling to the

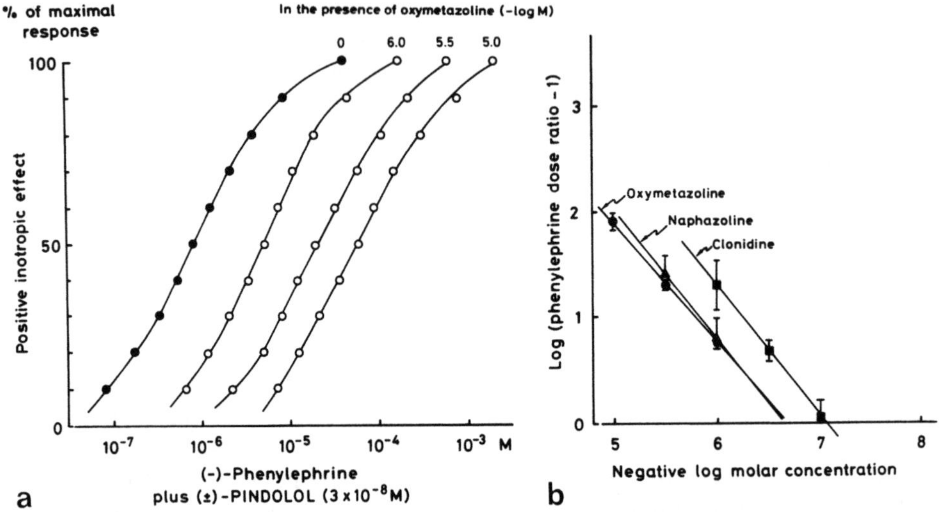

Fig. 1 a, b. Competitive antagonism by α-agonists (oxymetazoline, naphazoline and clonidine) of the positive inotropic effect of (−)-phenylephrine mediated by α-adrenoceptors, in the presence of 3×10^{-8} *M* (±)-pindolol in isolated rabbit papillary muscle. Stimulation frequency, 1 Hz; temperature, 37 °C. **a** Influence of various concentrations of oxymetazoline in the presence of (±)-pindolol; **b** relation between log (phenylephrine dose ratio −1) and the negative logarithm of the molar concentration of α-agonists has been plotted using the method of Arunlakshana and Schild (1959). The plot gave linear relationships with slope of −1.14 (oxymetazoline), −1.23 (naphazoline) and −1.24 (clonidine). The regression lines intersected the abscissa at the pA_2-values of 6.67 (oxymetazoline), 6.65 (naphazoline) and 7.05 (clonidine; modified from Schümann and Endoh 1976, by permission of the publisher)

biochemical process that occurs after the binding of sympathomimetic amines to the receptive site is different from that in other α_1-mediated systems. Thus, oxymetazoline and naphazoline (and clonidine) are capable of binding to the myocardial α-adrenoceptor site, but are not able to initiate the subsequent biochemical process, as a result of which they behave as competitive antagonists or partial agonists.

Differential Mechanisms of α- and β-Adrenoceptor-Mediated Actions

Cyclic AMP Metabolism

As was described briefly in the introduction, it has been established that the positive inotropic action of sympathomimetic amines induced by β-adrenoceptor stimulation is mediated by the production of cyclic AMP. In isolated rabbit papillary muscle, accumulation of cyclic AMP in the tissue precedes the increase in the force of contraction (Fig. 2). In contrast to β-stimulation, pure α-stimulation does not lead to a change in the cyclic AMP level of the tissue (Fig. 3).

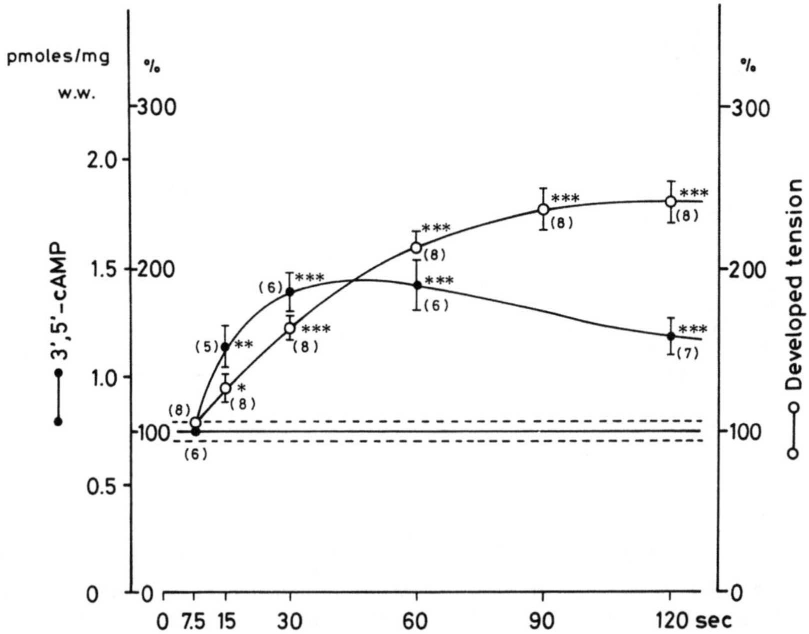

Fig. 2. Time course of the effects of 3×10^{-7} *M* (–)-isoprenaline on the cyclic AMP level and force developed in the isolated rabbit papillary muscle. Stimulation frequency, 0.5 Hz; temperature, 37 °C. *Abscissae,* time after the administration of (–)-isoprenaline in s; *solid horizontal line with broken lines,* control cyclic AMP level (means ± SE; $n = 11$) before the administration of (–)-isoprenaline. $^*P < 0.01$; $^{**}P < 0.005$; $^{***}P < 0.001$ vs the respective controls before the administration of (–)-isoprenaline. 100% of developed tension, 1.99 ± 0.15 m*N* ($n = 8$). Numbers of experiments in *parentheses* (from Schümann et al. 1975, by permission of the publisher)

Since the tissue cyclic AMP level is modulated in a complex manner by the balance of the activation of adenylate cyclase and cyclic AMP phosphodiesterase (PDE) [the activities of which may be also regulated by the intracellular Ca^{++} concentration (Tada et al. 1975; Dumont et al. 1984)], the lack of cyclic AMP accumulation during myocardial α-adrenoceptor stimulation does not necessarily rule out changes in cyclic AMP metabolism. If the activities of both enzymes were increased to a similar extent, the tissue cyclic AMP level might not change.

As originally postulated by Sutherland et al. (1968), inhibition of cyclic AMP PDE activity provides a useful means of resolving this difficulty. Theophylline and papaverine, prototypes of cyclic AMP PDE inhibitors, enhance the positive inotropic action and accumulation of cyclic AMP induced by β-adrenoceptor stimulation, but not the positive inotropic action mediated by α-adrenoceptors or produced by elevating the extracellular Ca^{++} concentration (which also does not cause the accumulation of cyclic AMP; Endoh et al. 1976a) (Fig. 4).

Muscarinic cholinergic receptor agonists provide another useful pharmacological tool for differentiating the cyclic AMP-mediated positive inotropic action from the cyclic AMP-independent action in mammalian ventricular myocardium. The muscarinic agonist has little effect on either the basal force of contraction or the cy-

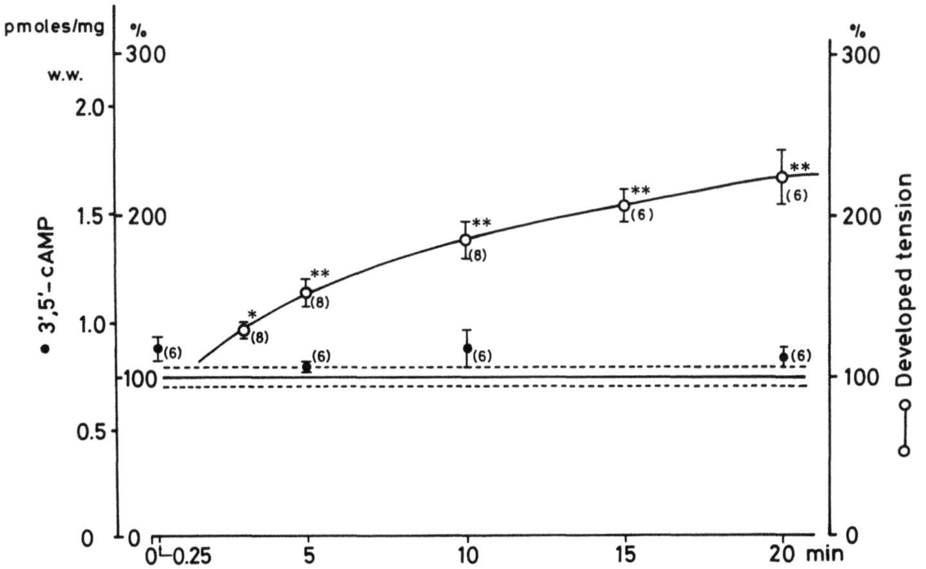

Fig. 3. Time course of the effects of 10^{-4} *M* methoxamine on the cyclic AMP level and tension developed in the isolated rabbit papillary muscle. Stimulation frequency, 0.5 Hz; temperature, 37 °C. *Abscissae*, time after the administration of methoxamine in min. * $P<0.01$, ** $P<0.001$ vs the respective controls of the cyclic AMP level and developed tension. 100% of developed tension, 1.90 ± 0.28 mN ($n=8$). Number of experiments in *parentheses* (from Schümann et al. 1975, by permission of the publisher)

clic AMP-independent positive inotropic actions of calcium, cardiac glycosides or Bay k 8644 (a calcium channel agonist). However, muscarinic cholinergic receptor agonists are capable of inhibiting effectively any actions mediated by cyclic AMP, such as those of β-adrenoceptor agonists, PDE inhibitors (papaverine, theophylline, caffeine and 3-isobutyl-1-methyl-xanthine), histamine, glucagon (Watanabe and Besch 1975; Endoh 1979, 1980; Biegon et al. 1980), cholera toxin (Pappano et al. 1982; Endoh et al. 1984), forskolin and various new inotropic agents (Macleod 1985; Endoh et al. 1986). As shown in Fig. 5, carbachol, a muscarinic agonist, inhibits the positive inotropic action of (—)-isoproterenol or (—)-phenylephrine mediated by β-adrenoceptors in the presence of phentolamine, an α-antagonist, but does not reduce the positive inotropic action of (—)-phenylephrine mediated by α-adrenoceptors in the presence of a β-antagonist, (±)-pindolol.

Adenosine is also capable of differentiating mechanisms in mammalian ventricular myocardium which are β-mediated (cyclic AMP-dependent) from those which are α-mediated (cyclic AMP-independent). Adenosine inhibits the β-mediated positive inotropic action of (—)-isoproterenol, but does not at all affect the α-mediated action of (—)-phenylephrine in the rabbit papillary muscle (Fig. 6).

The specific inhibitory action of muscarinic agonists and adenosine on cyclic AMP-mediated positive inotropic actions may involve multiple mechanisms: (a) a reduction of cyclic AMP generation by inhibition of adenylate cyclase activity through modulation of the inhibitory guanine nucleotide regulatory protein (N_i) (Murad et al. 1962; Ui 1984; Jakobs et al. 1984; Ui et al. 1984); (b) activation of

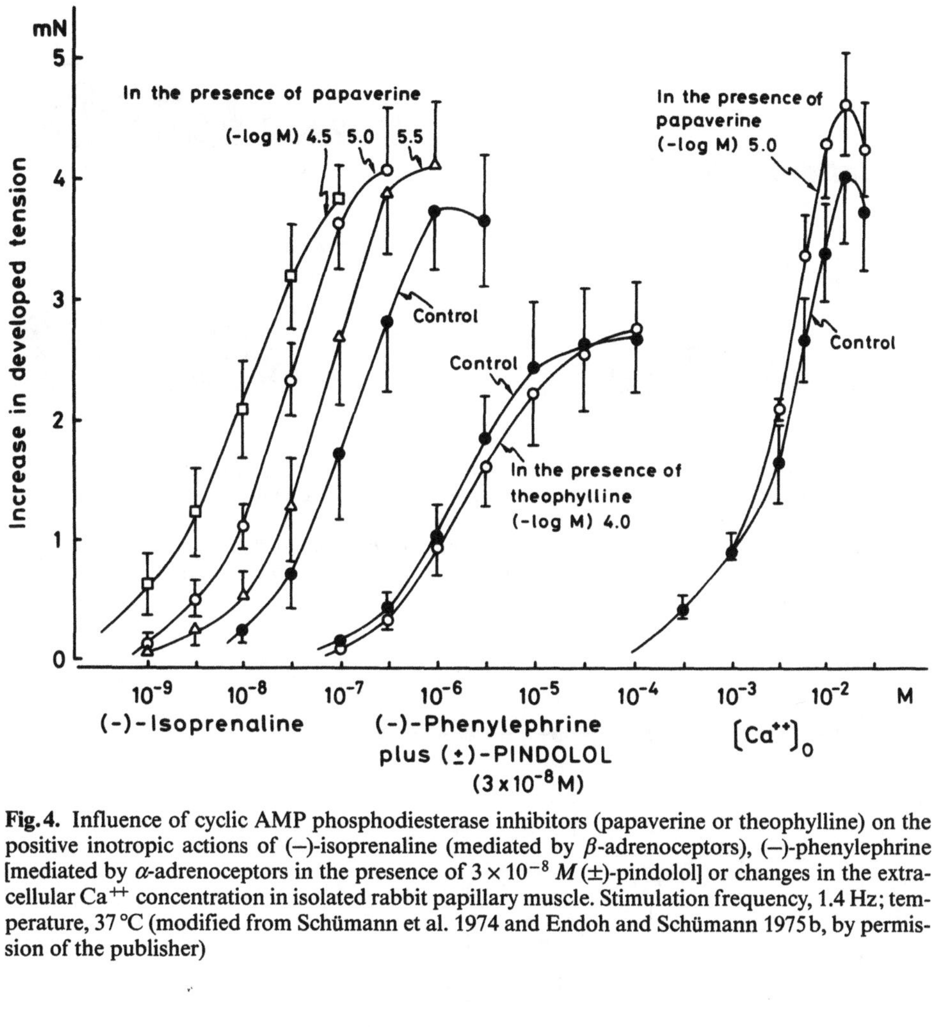

Fig. 4. Influence of cyclic AMP phosphodiesterase inhibitors (papaverine or theophylline) on the positive inotropic actions of (–)-isoprenaline (mediated by β-adrenoceptors), (–)-phenylephrine [mediated by α-adrenoceptors in the presence of 3×10^{-8} M (±)-pindolol] or changes in the extracellular Ca^{++} concentration in isolated rabbit papillary muscle. Stimulation frequency, 1.4 Hz; temperature, 37 °C (modified from Schümann et al. 1974 and Endoh and Schümann 1975b, by permission of the publisher)

PDE activity via muscarinic receptor stimulation (Van Sande et al. 1977; Barber et al. 1980; Meeker and Harden 1982) and (c) the dephosphorylation of functional proteins that have been phosphorylated through activation of cyclic AMP-dependent protein kinases (Biegon et al. 1980; Pappano et al. 1982; Iwasa and Hosey 1983; Böhm et al. 1984). It is not yet clear which of these mechanisms play important physiological roles in the working myocardium of various animal species. There seem to be substantial species differences in the relative contributions of the various mechanisms: the second and third mechanisms may explain the observations in certain animal species, but remain to be examined experimentally in the myocardium (for a more detailed discussion, see Endoh et al. 1984, 1985, 1986).

Whatever the subcellular mechanisms of the inhibitory actions induced by muscarinic agonists and adenosine, these mechanisms indicate quite clearly that the positive inotropic actions of sympathomimetic amines mediated by myocardial α-adrenoceptors do not involve changes in cyclic AMP metabolism.

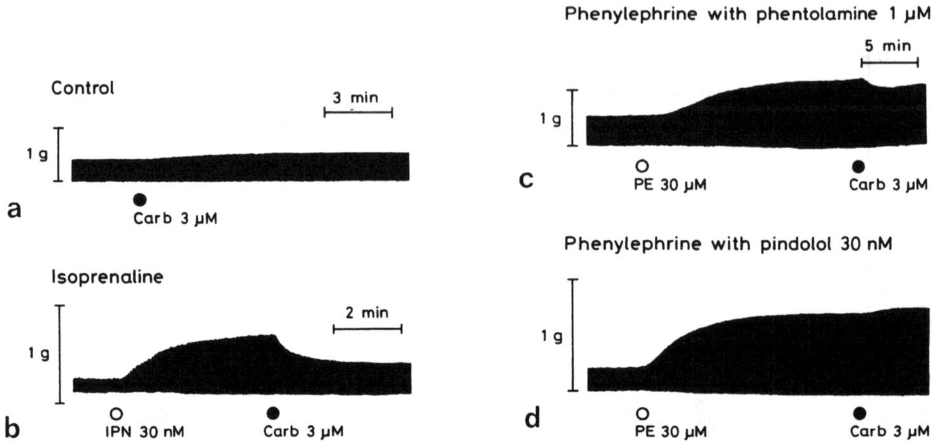

Fig. 5 a–d. Influence of the muscarinic agonist carbachol (3×10^{-6} *M; Carb*) on the β- or α-adrenoceptor-mediated positive inotropic actions in isolated rabbit papillary muscle. Stimulation frequency, 0.5 Hz; temperature, 37 °C. **a** Carbachol alone; **b** in the presence of 3×10^{-8} *M* (–)-isoprenaline *(IPN);* **c** in the presence of 3×10^{-5} *M* (–)-phenylephrine *(PE)* and 10^{-6} *M* phentolamine and **d** in the presence of *PE* and 3×10^{-8} *M* (±)-pindolol (from Endoh and Motomura 1979, by permission of the publisher)

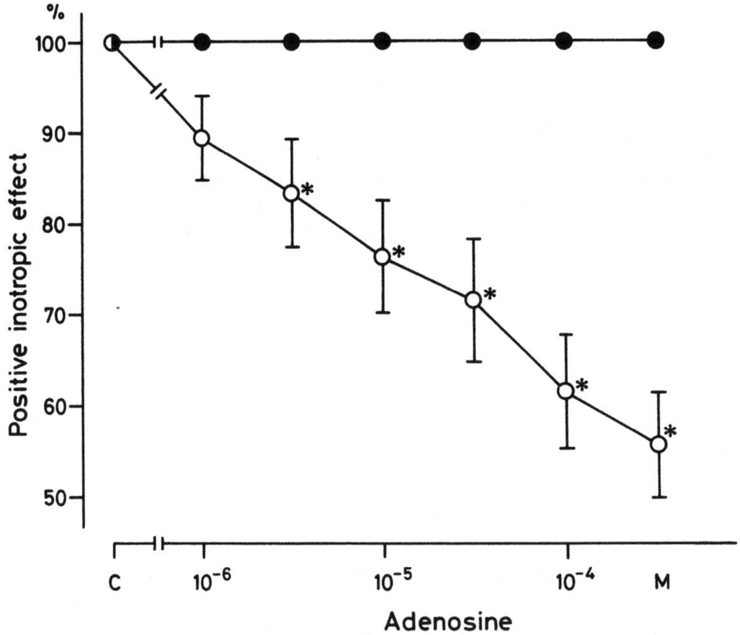

Fig. 6. Influence of adenosine on β- or α-adrenoceptor-mediated positive inotropic actions in isolated rabbit papillary muscle. Stimulation frequency, 0.5 Hz; temperature, 37 °C. The increase in the tension developed just prior to the administration of adenosine was taken as 100% *(C).* ●—●, phenylephrine with pindolol ($n = 4$); ○—○, isoprenaline with phentolamine ($n = 5$); * $P < 0.05$ vs the control value (from Endoh and Yamashita 1980, by permission of the publisher)

Relaxant Effect

β-Adrenoceptor stimulation accelerates the relaxation of heart muscle partly by increasing the rate of Ca^{++} sequestration [through phosphorylation of the sarcoplasmic reticulum membrane protein phospholamban (Tada and Katz 1982)] and partly by decreasing the Ca^{++} sensitivity of the thin filaments (Winegrad 1984). Together, these are known as the relaxant effect of β-stimulation (Tsien 1977). In the presence of α-adrenoceptor blockade, (–)-phenylephrine abbreviates the contraction by stimulating β-adrenoceptors (Fig. 7 A), and in the presence of the β-adrenoceptor blockade, it prolongs the contraction by α-stimulation (Fig. 7 B). This differential effect of (–)-phenylephrine on the relaxation phase has been observed in the myo-

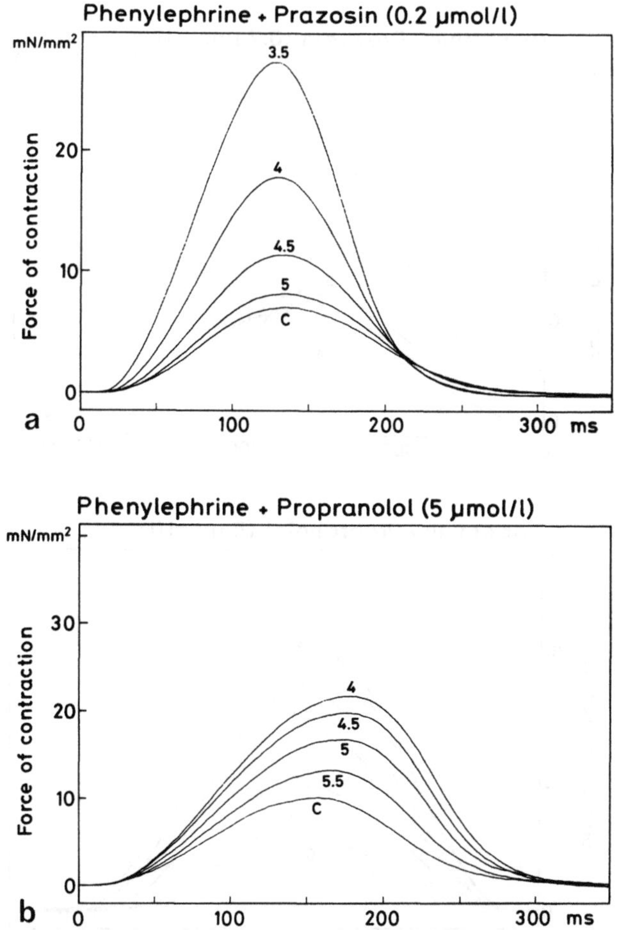

Fig. 7 a, b. Influence of (–)-phenylephrine on the time course and intensity of contraction in the isolated rabbit papillary muscle. Stimulation frequency, 1 Hz; temperature, 37 °C. **a** In the presence of 2×10^{-7} *M* prazosin; **b** in the presence of 5×10^{-6} *M* (±)-propranolol. Numbers adjacent to curves indicate $-\log M$ concentration of (–)-phenylephrine; *C*, control (M. Endoh and T. Yanagisawa, unpublished data)

cardium of the guinea pig (Ledda et al. 1975), rat (Osnes et al. 1978), cat (Scholz 1980) and rabbit (Aass et al. 1983).

In the rabbit papillary muscle, dopamine produces its positive inotropic action through both α- and β-adrenoceptors in the same concentration range. Although we earlier reported that a β-adrenoceptor antagonist, (±)-pindolol, $10^{-8}-3\times10^{-8}$ *M* did not affect the inotropic action of dopamine in the rabbit papillary muscle (Endoh et al. 1976b; Schümann et al. 1977; Brodde et al. 1980), that may have occurred because inadequate β-blockade was achieved with (±)-pindolol in the concentrations used. More recently, we have found that in the presence of a more potent β-adrenoceptor antagonist [(±)-bupranolol], the positive inotropic action of dopamine (and its action on the amplitude of the aequorin signals described later in the next section) was decreased and became very similar to the action of

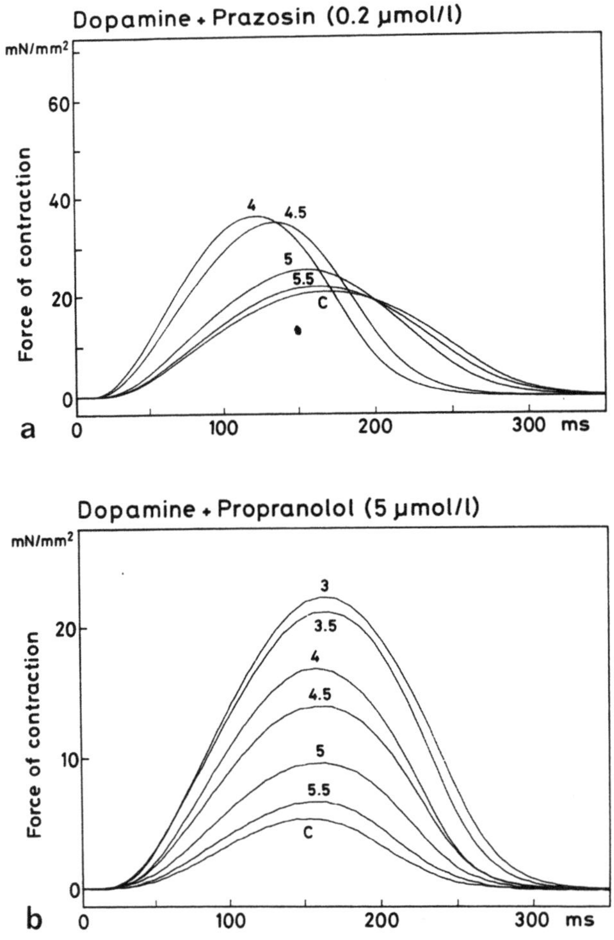

Fig. 8 a, b. Influence of dopamine on the time course and intensity of contraction in isolated rabbit papillary muscle. Stimulation frequency, 1 Hz; temperature, 37 °C. **a** In the presence of 2×10^{-7} *M* prazosin; **b** in the presence of 5×10^{-6} *M* (±)-propranolol. Numbers adjacent to curves indicate $-\log$ *M* concentration of dopamine; *C*, control (M. Endoh and T. Yanagisawa, unpublished data)

(–)-phenylephrine mediated by α-adrenoceptors (Endoh and Blinks 1986). Figure 8 shows the concentration-dependent effects of dopamine mediated by β- (A) or α-adrenoceptors (B) on the time course and strength of contraction of the rabbit papillary muscle. In the presence of 2×10^{-7} *M* prazosin, dopamine abbreviates the duration and time-to-peak of contraction by stimulating β-adrenoceptors (Fig. 8 A), while in the presence of 5×10^{-6} *M* (±)-propranolol it prolongs the contractions slightly by stimulating α-adrenoceptors (Fig. 8 B).

Whether or not myocardial α-adrenoceptors play a role in producing the positive inotropic effect of noradrenaline in mammalian ventricular myocardium has been a matter of controversy. We were not able to detect an α-adrenoceptor-mediated effect of (–)-noradrenaline in the rabbit papillary muscle in the presence of 10^{-8}

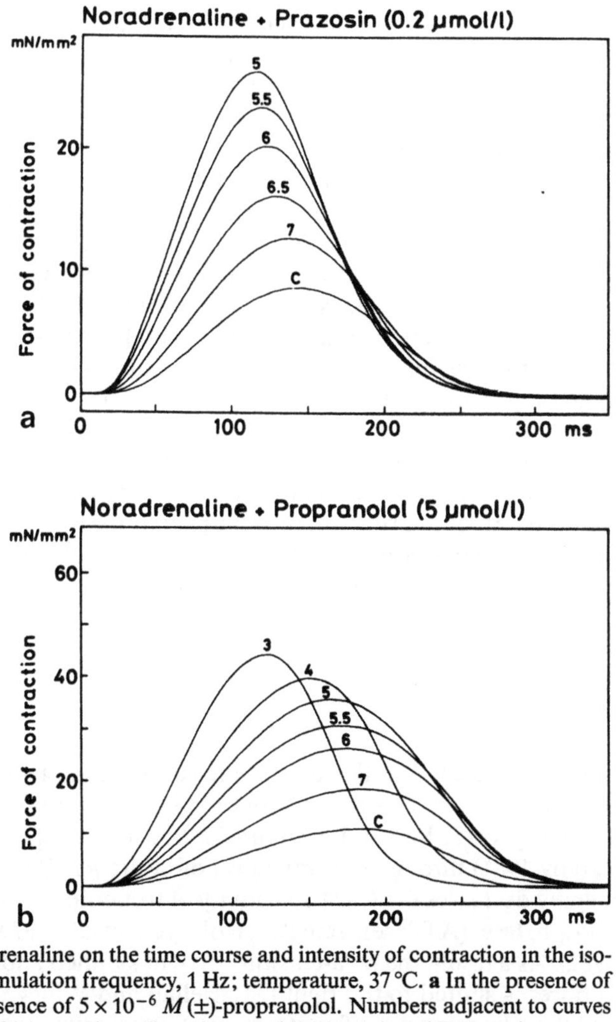

Fig. 9 a, b. Influence of (–)-noradrenaline on the time course and intensity of contraction in the isolated rabbit papillary muscle. Stimulation frequency, 1 Hz; temperature, 37 °C. **a** In the presence of 2×10^{-7} *M* prazosin; **b** in the presence of 5×10^{-6} *M* (±)-propranolol. Numbers adjacent to curves indicate $-\log M$ concentration of (–)-noradrenaline; *C*, control (M. Endoh and T. Yanagisawa, unpublished data)

or 3×10^{-8} M(±)-pindolol at 37 °C (Schümann et al. 1974; Endoh et al. 1976b); however, Aass et al. (1983) reported that (–)-noradrenaline increased the force of contraction on the same preparation in the presence of 5×10^{-6} M (±)-propranolol at 32 °C. This effect was inhibited by the α_1-antagonist prazosin. In an effort to determine the reason for this discrepancy, we recently repeated our earlier experiments in the rabbit papillary muscle using 5×10^{-6} M (±)-propranolol to achieve β-adrenoceptor blockade. Figure 9 shows the positive inotropic action of (–)-noradrenaline in the presence of 2×10^{-7} M prazosin (A) and 5×10^{-6} M (±)-propranolol (B) at 37 °C in the rabbit papillary muscle. In the presence of prazosin, (–)-noradrenaline in each concentration abbreviated the duration of contraction (Fig. 9 A). On the other hand, in the presence of 5×10^{-6} M (±)-propranolol, (–)-noradrenaline in concentrations up to 3×10^{-6} M increased the force of contraction with little change in the time course of contraction; in concentrations of 10^{-5} M and higher, it abbreviated the duration and time-to-peak of contraction (Fig. 9 B). It is evident, therefore, that our failure to detect the α-mediated effect of (–)-noradrenaline in the earlier study was due to the use of (±)-pindolol as a β-antagonist: the β-blockade achieved by 10^{-8} to 3×10^{-8} M (±)-pindolol was inadequate and readily overcome by increasing the concentration of an agonist with the potent β-adrenoceptor stimulatory activity of (–)-noradrenaline.

Another factor may have helped to obscure the expression of weak α-adrenoceptor stimulation by (–)-noradrenaline in the presence of (±)-pindolol. (±)-Pindolol is a weak partial agonist at the β-adrenoceptor, and in at least some species (e.g. dog, see Nayler 1972; cat, see Kaumann and Blinks 1980) has positive inotropic effects in the range of concentrations used in the former study. In some preparations of rabbit papillary muscle, 3×10^{-8} M(±)-pindolol produced a slight positive inotropic action (though the effect was not statistically significant on the average). This weak intrinsic β-mediated activity of (±)-pindolol might have tended to obscure the weak α-mediated action of (–)-noradrenaline. On the other hand, (±)-propranolol (5×10^{-6} M) decreased the force of contraction to 53.4% ± 2.4% ($n=4$) of the basal level prior to the administration of propranolol. This cardiodepressant action of (±)-propranolol (mainly the result of a non-specific action of the compound) may have produced a condition in which the weak α-mediated action of (–)-noradrenaline is more easily expressed.

Ca^{++} Sensitivity

Available evidence indicates that the stimulation of β-adrenoceptors catalyzes the phosphorylation of a protein (troponin I) of the thin filaments (England 1975; Cole and Perry 1975; Ray and England 1976; Mope et al. 1980; Stull 1980; Bárány and Bárány 1981) through the activation of cyclic AMP-dependent protein kinase and thereby decreases the Ca^{++} sensitivity of troponin C and myofibrillar adenosine triphosphatase (ATPase) activity (Holroyde et al. 1979; Yamamoto and Ohtsuki 1982). As a result, the pCa-tension curve of skinned and hyperpermeable myocardial fibres is shifted to the right (McClellan and Winegrad 1978; Herzig et al. 1981) and the relaxation rate of contraction of intact myocardial cell preparations is accelerated (Solaro 1982; Demaille et al. 1983; Katz 1983; Winegrad 1984; Blinks and

Endoh 1986). Evidence for this mechanism has been obtained in biochemical experiments (in broken cell and perfused heart preparations) and in skinned and hyperpermeable myocardial fibres as described above. The physiological significance of the mechanism in intact myocardial cells has been examined more directly by the application of calcium-sensitive microelectrodes (Marban et al. 1980) and of the calcium-sensitive bioluminescent protein aequorin (Blinks 1984).

In isolated rabbit papillary muscles in which multiple superficial cells had been microinjected with aequorin, the force developed and the aequorin light signal are altered in parallel by changing the extracellular calcium concentration (Fig. 10, left panel). The relation of changes in force developed to changes in the amplitude of the aequorin signals [(peak light)$^{1/2.5}$] is essentially linear (Fig. 10, right panel). It seems reasonable to assume that in any given preparation, the slope of the line will vary with changes in the Ca^{++} sensitivity of the contractile apparatus induced by inotropic agents. It has been shown that the relation becomes shallower during the stimulation of β-adrenoceptors in the cat (Allen and Kurihara 1980; Blinks et al. 1982; Morgan and Blinks 1982; J.P. Morgan and K.G. Morgan 1984) and rabbit papillary muscle (Endoh and Blinks 1986).

Figure 11 shows the effects of (–)-phenylephrine in the presence of 10^{-7} *M* (±)-bupranolol on aequorin signals and isometric contractions in an aequorin-injected rabbit papillary muscle. There is an increase in the amplitude of the aequorin signals during the α-adrenoceptor-mediated positive inotropic action, but the increase in the amplitude of the aequorin signals is much less prominent than that

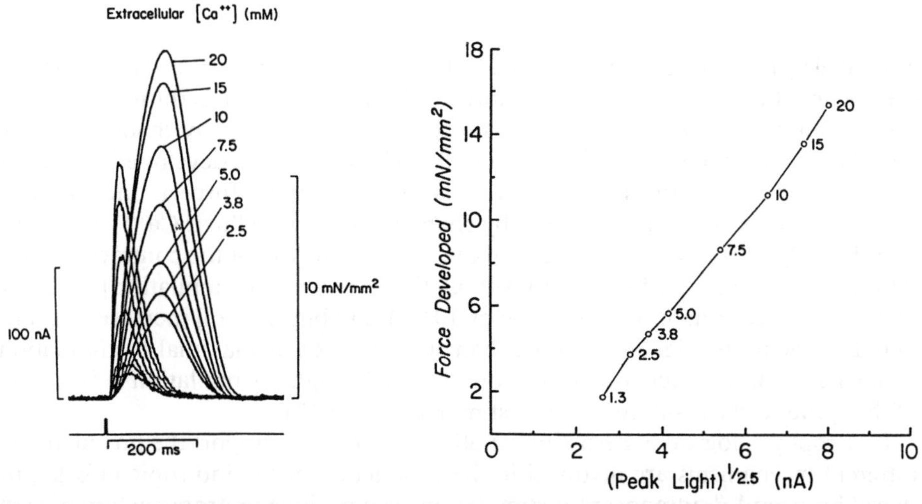

Fig. 10. Effects of altering the extracellular calcium concentration on aequorin signals (intracellular Ca^{++} transients, *noisy tracings*) and contractions in an isolated rabbit papillary muscle (length, 6.5 mm; cross-sectional area, 0.74 mm^2), in which the superficial cells had been microinjected with the calcium-sensitive bioluminescent protein aequorin. Stimulation frequency, 1 Hz; temperature, 37.5 °C. *Left panel,* signal-averaged records, each from 128 successive contractions with aequorin signals and isometric contractions superimposed. *Numbers* indicate the extracellular Ca^{++} concentration (m*M*). *Right panel,* the relation between the force developed and (peak aequorin signal)$^{1/2.5}$ (M. Endoh and J.R. Blinks, unpublished data)

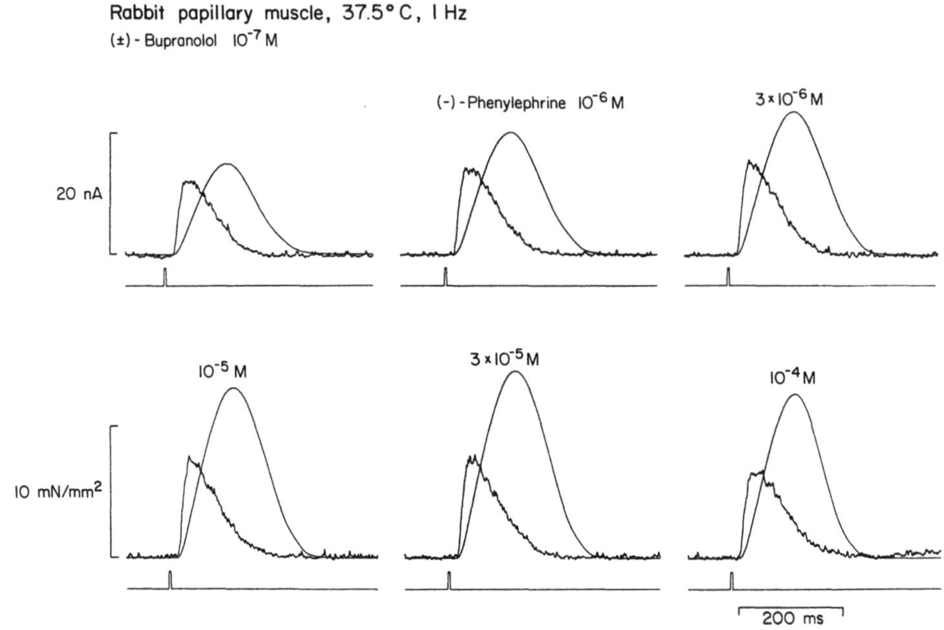

Fig. 11. Effects of (–)-phenylephrine mediated via α-adrenoceptors in the presence of 10^{-7} *M* (±)-bupranolol on aequorin signals and contractions in isolated rabbit papillary muscle. Signal-averaged records from 128 successive contractions with aequorin signals *(noisy tracings)* and isometric contractions superimposed. Stimulation frequency, 1 Hz; temperature, 37.5 °C (M. Endoh and J. R. Blinks, unpublished data)

produced by (–)-isoprenaline (cf. Fig. 15). In fact, for a given increase in the force of contraction, the increase in the amplitude of the aequorin signals during α-adrenoceptor stimulation is much less than when the force is increased by changing the extracellular calcium concentration. That is, the relation of force developed to the amplitude of the aequorin signal is much steeper when the force is increased by α-stimulation than when it is altered by changing the extracellular Ca^{++} concentration (Fig. 12). This finding suggests that the Ca^{++} sensitivity of the contractile apparatus is *increased* by α-adrenoceptor stimulation. Maximal α-stimulation [produced by (–)-phenylephrine in the presence of 10^{-7} *M* (±)-bupranolol] increases the amplitude of aequorin signals no more than 10% as much as maximal β-stimulation, while the maximum increase in force developed through α-stimulation is 50%–60% of that produced by β-adrenoceptor stimulation (Fig. 13).

Electrophysiological experiments in other species also support the postulate that different mechanisms are involved in the production of the inotropic effects produced by α- and β-adrenoceptor stimulation. The positive inotropic action of sympathomimetic amines mediated via α-adrenoceptors is not associated with detectable changes in the Ca^{++}-dependent slow response action potential in guinea pig papillary muscle (Ledda et al. 1980; Sanchez-Chapula 1981). In bovine ventricular trabeculae, it was found that for a given increase in developed force, the maximum rate of rise of the slow response was increased much less by α-stimulation than by β-stimulation (Brückner and Scholz 1984).

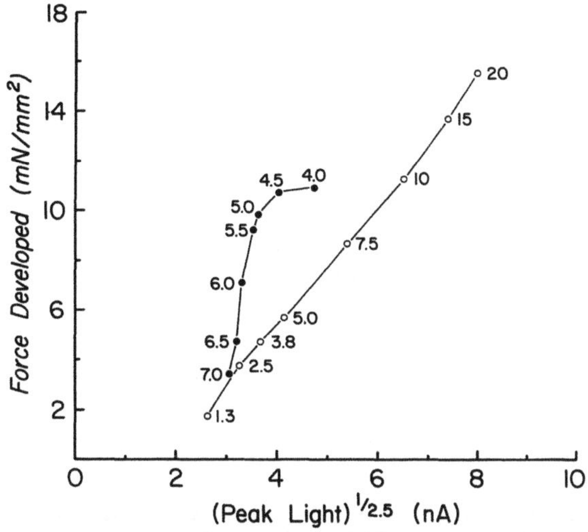

Fig. 12. Relation of force developed to (peak aequorin signal)$^{1/2.5}$ during stimulation of α-adrenoceptors in comparison with the relation when contractility was varied by changing the extracellular Ca^{++} concentration in the same isolated rabbit papillary muscle. Stimulation frequency, 1 Hz; temperature, 37.5 °C. ●, (–)-phenylephrine (–log *M*)+(±)-bupranolol 10^{-6} *M;* ○, extracellular [Ca^{++}] (m*M*) (Endoh and Blinks 1986)

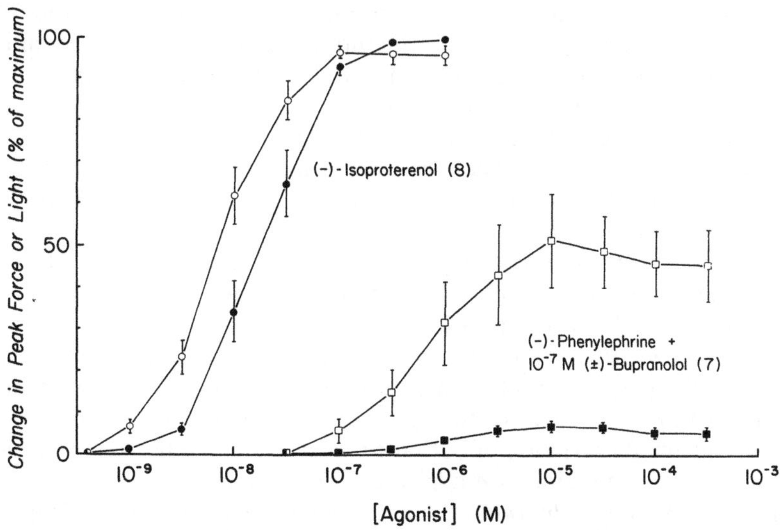

Fig. 13. Concentration-response curves for (–)-isoprenaline and for (–)-phenylephrine [in the presence of 10^{-7} *M*(±)-bupranolol] in rabbit papillary muscle. Increases in the amplitude of the aequorin signals and of the force developed are plotted as percentages of the maximum increase obtained in response to (–)-isoprenaline. ○ □, force developed; ● ■, peak light (from Endoh and Blinks 1986)

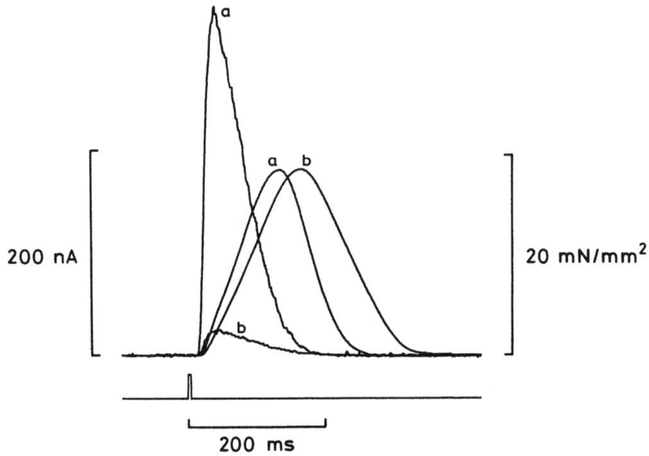

Fig. 14. Influence of 10^{-4} *M* dopamine on aequorin signals and isometric contractions in the aequorin-injected rabbit papillary muscle in the absence *(a)* and presence *(b)* of 10^{-6} *M* (±)-bupranolol. Muscle length, 8 mm; cross-sectional area, 0.95 mm^2; stimulation frequency, 1 Hz; temperature, 37.5 °C. Signal-averaged records of 64 (dopamine alone) and 128 [dopamine + (±)-bupranolol] successive contractions superimposed (M. Endoh and J. R. Blinks, unpublished data)

Since dopamine produces its positive inotropic action both through *α*- and *β*-adrenoceptors in the same concentration range (see above), the differential effects of *α*- and *β*-stimulation on the intracellular Ca^{++} transients and contraction are most clearly seen when this compound is administered in the aequorin-injected rabbit papillary muscle. Figure 14 shows the influence of (±)-bupranolol on the effects of 10^{-4} *M* dopamine. (±)-Bupranolol markedly reduced the amplitude of the aequorin signals (which had been previously increased by dopamine) and prolonged the duration of contraction (which had been abbreviated previously by dopamine). In this particular experiment, the increase in peak tension produced by dopamine was the same in the presence and absence of bupranolol, though the contractions in the presence of *β*-blockade were of longer duration and were associated with much smaller aequorin signals (*b* in Fig. 14).

The changes in the time course of contraction and aequorin signals also lend support to the postulate that *α*-adrenoceptor stimulation leads to an increase in the Ca^{++}-affinity of the contractile apparatus. Stimulation of *β*-adrenoceptors leads to a prominent abbreviation of both the contractions and the aequorin signals. On the other hand, stimulation of *α*-adrenoceptors *prolongs* the contraction (as also shown in Figs. 7-9), but *abbreviates* the aequorin signals (Endoh and Blinks 1984, 1986; Blinks and Endoh 1986). This finding can be explained if the Ca^{++} affinity of troponin C is increased: less Ca^{++} is available for aequorin bioluminescence because more Ca^{++} is bound longer to troponin C.

In isolated rabbit papillary muscle, carbachol by itself does not influence the aequorin signal or the isometric contraction, but antagonizes the effects of (–)-isoprenaline. In the presence of 3×10^{-6} *M* carbachol, the increase in the amplitude of the aequorin signals and of the contractions produced by (–)-isoproterenol was markedly attenuated (Fig. 15 A, B). On the other hand, carbachol has no effect on

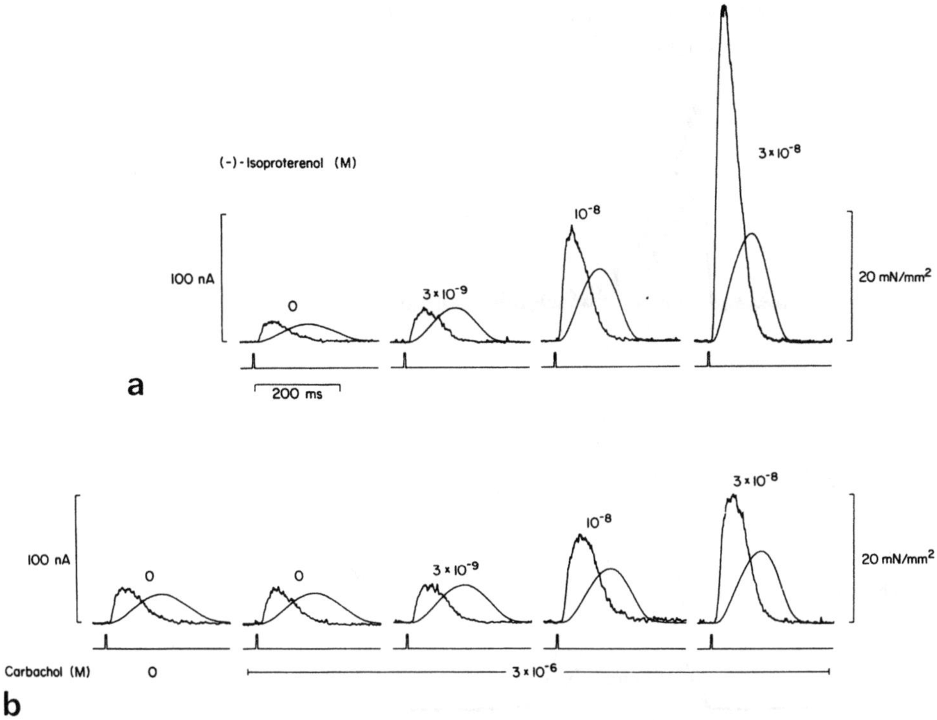

Fig. 15 a, b. Influence of carbachol (3×10^{-6} *M*) on β-adrenoceptor-mediated responses of the aequorin signal and isometric contraction in an aequorin-injected rabbit papillary muscle. Muscle length, 5.5 mm; cross-sectional area, 0.50 mm^2; stimulation frequency, 1 Hz; temperature, 37.5 °C. **a** (–)-isoprenaline alone; **b** (–)-isoprenaline in the presence of 3×10^{-6} *M* carbachol. Signal-averaged records from 64 successive contractions superimposed (M. Endoh and J. R. Blinks, unpublished data)

aequorin signals or contractions which have been increased by α-adrenoceptor stimulation (Fig. 16). This is consistent with the findings of previous studies on the contractions of rabbit papillary muscle (Endoh and Motomura 1979; Inui et al. 1982).

Other Interventions

The positive inotropic actions of sympathomimetic amines mediated by myocardial α- and β-adrenoceptors are influenced differently by a variety of experimental interventions. These include changes in the frequency of contraction or changes in experimental temperature (Endoh and Schümann 1975 a; Endoh et al. 1975, 1977), alterations in the level of thyroid hormone (Nakashima et al. 1971, 1973; Wagner and Brodde 1978; Gross and Lues 1985) and administration of the calcium entry blocker D600 (Endoh et al. 1975; Ledda et al. 1975).

An example of the differential effects of temperature on the α- and β-mediated actions of (–)-phenylephrine is shown in Fig. 17. Lowering the temperature from

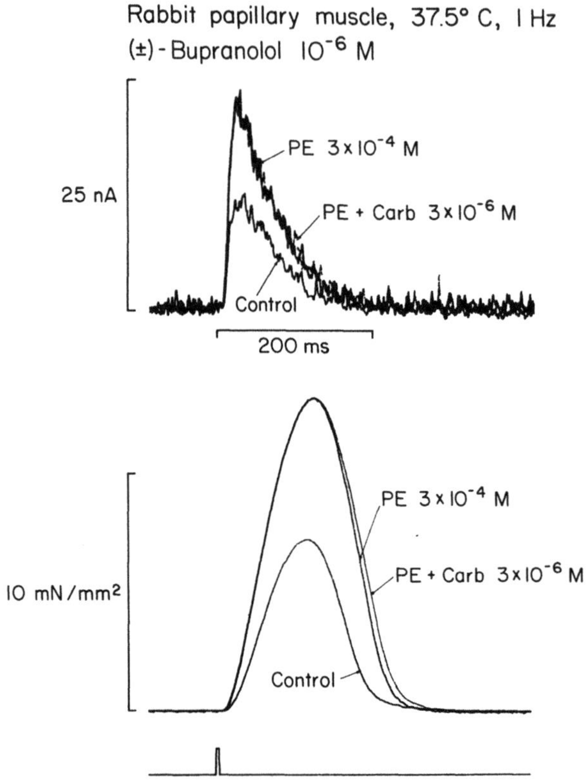

Fig. 16. Influence of carbachol *(Carb;* 3×10^{-6} *M)* on α-adrenoceptor-mediated responses of the aequorin signal and isometric contraction in an aequorin-injected rabbit papillary muscle. Muscle length, 6.2 mm; cross-sectional area, 0.49 mm²; stimulation frequency, 1 Hz; temperature, 37.5 °C. Signal-averaged records from 256 successive contractions with aequorin signals *(upper panel)* and isometric contractions *(lower panel)* superimposed. *PE,* (−)-phenylephrine; 10^{-6} *M* (±)-bupranolol was present throughout (M. Endoh and J. R. Blinks, unpublished data)

37 °C to 32 °C shifted the concentration-response curves of both α- and β-mediated actions to the left to a similar extent, while raising the temperature from 37 °C to 42 °C influenced the β-mediated action only slightly, but markedly shifted the curve of the α-mediated action.

The mechanisms underlying these differential effects of diverse interventions on α- and β-mediated actions are not known, but several common features seem to be involved. Firstly, the facilitation of transmembrane Ca^{++} flux resulting from stimulation of α-adrenoceptors is much less than that induced by β-adrenoceptor stimulation when detected as the slow response (Miura et al. 1978) or slow inward current (Brückner and Scholz 1984) or as the intracellular calcium transient (Endoh and Blinks 1984, 1986).

Secondly, the number of α- and β-adrenoceptor binding sites has been shown to be regulated by the level of thyroid hormone. Hyperthyroid states increase the number of binding sites of β-adrenoceptors and reduce that of α-adrenoceptors; these

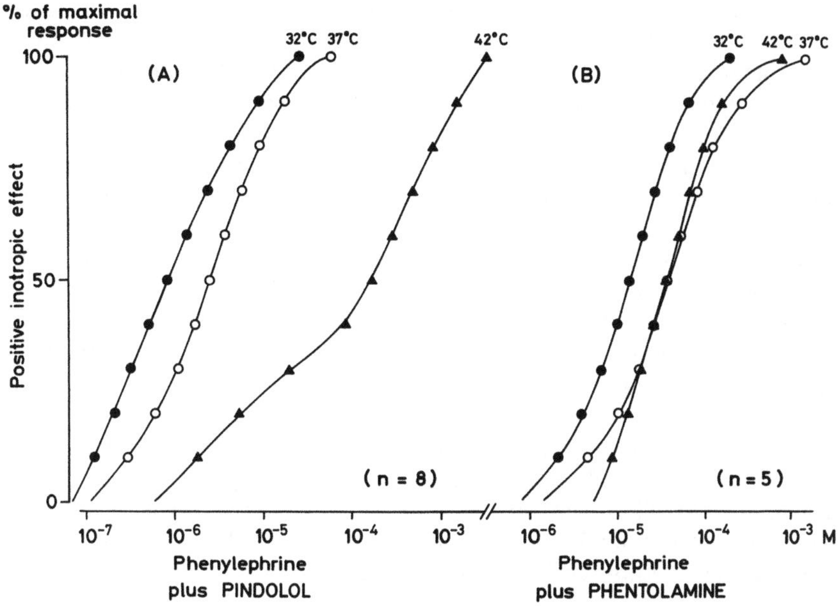

Fig. 17. Influence of temperature on the positive inotropic actions of (–)-phenylephrine mediated by α-adrenoceptors [in the presence of 3×10^{-8} *M* (±)-pindolol] **(A)** and mediated by β-adrenoceptors (in the presence of 10^{-6} *M* phentolamine) **(B)** in isolated rabbit papillary muscle. Stimulation frequency, 0.5 Hz (from Endoh et al. 1977, by permission of the publisher)

changes are consistent with the direction of modification of functional changes, i. e. enhancement of β-mediated actions and suppression of α-mediated actions in hyperthyroid states (Kunos 1977; Williams et al. 1977; Ciaraldi and Marinetti 1977; Hashimoto and Nakashima 1978; Sharma and Banerjee 1978; Tsai and Chen 1978; Williams and Lefkowitz 1979; McConnaughey et al. 1979).

On the other hand, the influence of hypothyroid states cannot be explained solely by changes in the number of adrenoceptor binding sites. The number of β-adrenoceptor binding sites and β-mediated actions are both decreased in hypothyroid states; however, while α-mediated actions are consistently enhanced in hypothyroid states, this change is associated with decreased (Ciaraldi and Marinetti 1977; McConnaughey et al. 1979) or unchanged (Williams and Lefkowitz 1979) numbers of α-adrenoceptor binding sites. Gross and Lues (1985 and this volume) carried out a large number of careful experiments in order to try to resolve this discrepancy and found that the number of α-binding sites is reduced in the hypothyroid state.

Thyroid states may also affect the regulation of myocardial contractility by β-adrenoceptor stimulation through modulation of the isozyme transition state of myosin in mammalian ventricular myocardium (Winegrad 1984). It has been shown that three isozymes of myosin (V1, V2 and V3) exist in rat ventricular myocardium; these migrate at different rates in polyacrylamide gels during electrophoresis in a pyrophosphate medium (Hoh et al. 1977). Hyperthyroidism states produced total transition of isozymes to V1 (the most rapidly migrating) with the highest Ca^{++}- and actin-activated ATPase activity in the rat (Hoh et al. 1977) and rabbit (Martin et al. 1982). Hypothyroidism caused a transition to the V3 isozyme (the most slowly migrating one), with the lowest ATPase activity in the rat (Hoh et al. 1977). In hyperpermeable rat myocardial cells, it has been shown that the cyclic AMP-dependent regulatory mechanism can recognize the different isozymes of myosin: cyclic AMP with theophylline and detergent produced an increase in maximum Ca^{++}-activated force that was proportional to the relative concentration of the V1 isozyme, but failed to increase the force in cells containing only the V3 myosin (Winegrad et al. 1983). On the other hand, the V3 myosin responds to α-stimulation in much the same way that the V1 myosin responds to β-stimulation (S. Winegrad et al., personal communication).

It has been known for some time that certain calcium entry blockers, such as verapamil, bind with high affinity to myocardial α-adrenoceptors (Glossman and Hornung 1980; Karliner et al. 1982; Motulsky et al. 1983). However, it was recently reported that D600, which has been used in functional studies to antagonize the α-mediated positive inotropic action (Endoh et al. 1975; Ledda et al. 1975), bound to the myocardial α-adrenoceptors only with relatively low affinity (Mukherjee et al. 1983; i.e. the IC_{50} for D600 to inhibit [^{3}H]prazosin binding is ca. 100 times higher than that for verapamil in the rabbit heart), suggesting that competition by this compound at the receptor level is not significant.

Perspectives on Functional Role and Putative Mediator of Myocardial α-Adrenoceptor Stimulation

In the ventricular myocardium of most mammalian species, adrenaline and noradrenaline produce their positive inotropic actions via stimulation of α-adrenoceptors in concentrations below those required to stimulate β-adrenoceptors (Schümann et al. 1974; Aass et al. 1983). While the β-adrenoceptor-mediated inotropic and chronotropic responses to endogenous catecholamines can be antagonized by vagal nerve stimulation, the α-adrenoceptor-mediated inotropic response cannot (Endoh and Motomura 1979; Inui et al. 1982). These observations suggest that myocardial α-adrenoceptors may play a physiologically significant role in the fine adjustment of myocardial contraction through the autonomic nervous system when small amounts of transmitters are released in order to match the cardiac function to momentary physical requirements.

The α-adrenoceptor-mediated positive inotropic action has been shown to be prominently dependent on the frequency of contraction and is less pronounced at high rates of contraction (for review, see Endoh 1982). In aequorin-injected atrial muscle, however, it is clear that (–)-phenylephrine is able to increase the intracellular calcium transient and to induce a positive inotropic effect via stimulation of α-adrenoceptors even at a rate of 4 Hz (Fig. 18). However, it is difficult to maintain a good contractile state in *isolated* ventricular muscle (either papillary muscle or trabecula) driven at such a high rate in an organ bath. It remains to be determined whether the frequency dependence of the α-mediated effect is a characteristic of the receptor-mediated process or whether an additional action of the compound contributes to the frequency dependence, as in the case of methoxamine (Imai 1961).

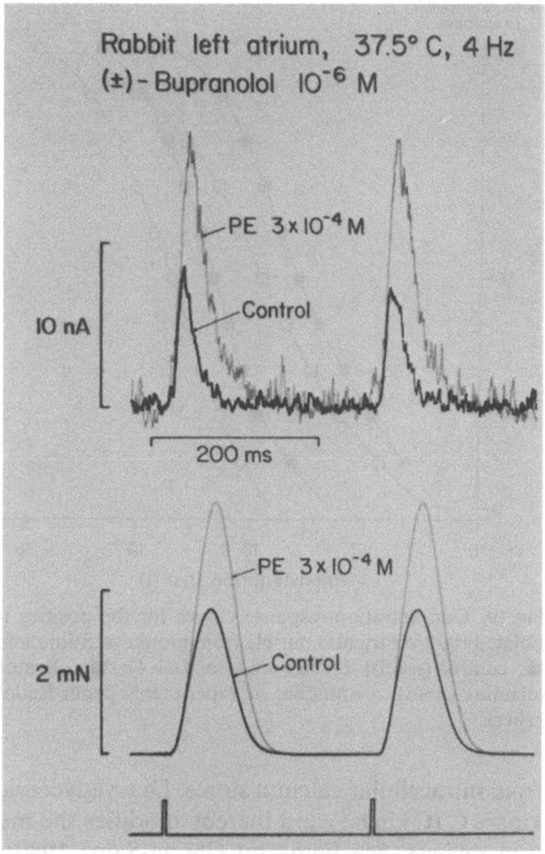

Fig. 18. α-Mediated effects of (–)-phenylephrine (3×10^{-4} *M*) on aequorin signals and isometric contractions in an isolated rabbit atrial trabecula. Frequency, 4 Hz; temperature, 37.5 °C; muscle length, 11 mm; cross-sectional area, 0.35 mm^2. Signal-averaged records from 258 successive contractions with superimposed aequorin signals in the *upper panel* and isometric contractions in the *lower panel*. 10^{-6} *M* (±)-bupranolol was present throughout (M. Endoh and J. R. Blinks, unpublished data)

In recent years, it has been shown that α-adrenoceptors are capable of mediating a positive inotropic effect in myocardium isolated from primates, including both monkeys (Fig. 19) and man (Schümann et al. 1978; Wagner et al. 1980; Brückner et al. 1984). These findings lend further support to the idea that α-adrenoceptors may play a functionally significant role in the regulation of human myocardial contractility in situ.

The subcellular process that couples α-adrenoceptor stimulation to augmentation of myocardial contractility has not yet been defined. Neither cyclic AMP nor cyclic GMP is involved (Brodde et al. 1978). It has been shown in recent years that the stimulation of myocardial α-adrenoceptors catalyzes polyphosphoinositide turnover in rat cultured myocardial cells (Uchida et al. 1982; Brown et al. 1985) and rat atria (Sekar and Roufogalis 1984). In other biological systems, inositol trisphosphate, one of the breakdown products of polyphosphoinositides, mobilizes calcium

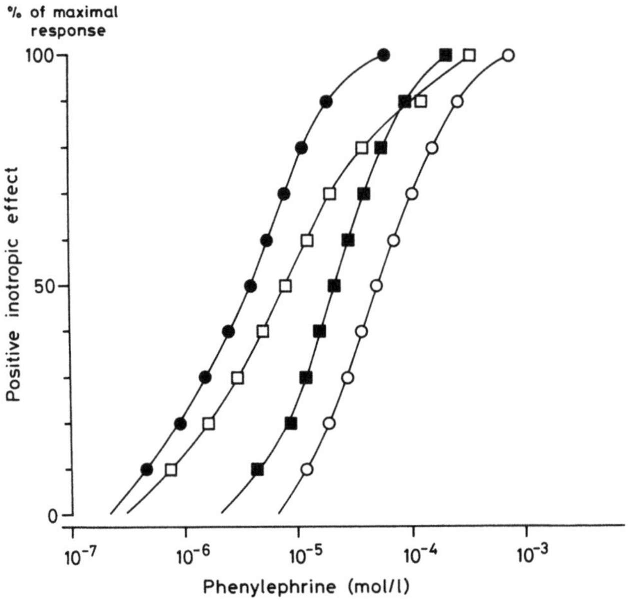

Fig. 19. Concentration-response curves for the positive inotropic effect of (–)-phenylephrine on isolated right ventricular muscle from monkeys. Stimulation frequency, 0.5 Hz; temperature, 37 °C. ●, control ($n=5$); □, (±)-pindolol ($n=4$); ■, phentolamine ($n=4$); ○, (±)-pindolol + phentolamine ($n=5$); n = number of experiments (from Endoh et al. 1982, by permission of the publisher)

from intracellular calcium stores. Diacylglycerol, another product, activates protein kinase C (C kinase) and thereby modifies the membrane transport of Ca^{++} (for recent reviews, see Fain and García-Sáinz 1980; Takai et al. 1981; Berridge 1981, 1984; Michell 1983; Nishizuka 1983; Berridge and Irvine 1984). Although it seems an attractive hypothesis that this system might be involved in mediating the physiological responses to myocardial α-adrenoceptor stimulation (Brückner et al. 1985; Brown et al. 1985), direct evidence for such involvement is so far lacking. In isolated canine cardiac sarcoplasmic reticulum, activation of C kinase and the resulting phosphorylation of a sarcoplasmic reticulum (SR) protein have recently been shown to be associated with a stimulation of Ca^{++} uptake (Movsesian et al. 1984). Stimulation of Ca^{++} uptake into the SR would be expected to bring about changes in the duration of contraction that are the opposite of those produced by stimulation of α-adrenoceptors in rabbit papillary muscle. However, as mentioned above, α-adrenoceptors do not play an important role in the positive inotropic action of sympathomimetic amines in the canine heart.

Conclusions

In mammalian myocardium, in addition to the predominant β-adrenoceptors, α-adrenoceptors are involved in the regulation of myocardial contractility. The α-

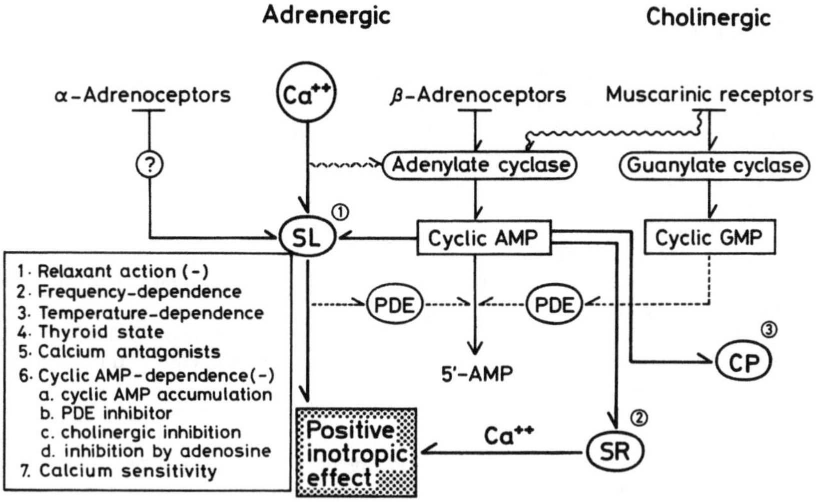

Fig. 20. Schematic diagram illustrating possible mechanisms of actions mediated via α- and β-adrenoceptors and of cholinergic stimulation in mammalian ventricular myocardium. Interventions that bring about differential responses of α- and β-adrenoceptor-mediated positive inotropic actions are listed in the *rectangle* at the left. β-Adrenoceptor stimulation causes the phosphorylation of functional proteins in the *1* sarcolemma *(SL); 2* sarcoplasmic reticulum *(SR)* and *3* contractile apparatus *(CP). Wavy (broken and solid) lines* indicate the potential inhibition of adenylate cyclase activity by elevation of the intracellular Ca^{++} concentration or by muscarinic receptor stimulation; *straight dotted lines* indicate the potential stimulation of cyclic AMP phosphodiesterase activity *(PDE)* by elevation of the intracellular Ca^{++} concentration or by muscarinic receptor stimulation. To avoid further complexity, the possible stimulation of phosphatase activity through muscarinic receptors has not been indicated

adrenoceptor-mediated positive inotropic action is initiated by the binding of sympathomimetic amine molecules to α_1-adrenoceptor binding sites on the outer surface of the myocardial cell membrane. The subcellular biochemical processes that result from myocardial α-adrenoceptor stimulation are much less well understood than those involved in the β-mediated process, but it is evident that the α-mediated action is elicited through a mechanism which is different from that of the β-mediated action in many respects. The interventions that modulate the α- and β-mediated positive inotropic actions in different ways are summarized in Fig. 20. The stimulation of myocardial α-adrenoceptors may increase the Ca^{++} sensitivity of the contractile apparatus, while β-adrenoceptor stimulation decreases the sensitivity. Current evidence favors the view that α-adrenoceptors play a functionally significant role in the regulation of myocardial contractility.

Acknowledgements. The author wishes to acknowledge that John R. Blinks, Mayo Foundation, and Teruyuki Yanagisawa, Tohoku University School of Medicine, have allowed the inclusion of some unpublished data as figures used in this paper. The author also thanks Dr. Blinks for reviewing and Toshiko Hashimoto for preparing the manuscript.

References

Aass H, Skomedal T, Osnes JB (1983) Demonstration of an alpha adrenoceptor-mediated inotropic effect of norepinephrine in rabbit papillary muscle. J Pharmacol Exp Ther 226: 572-578

Allen DG, Kurihara S (1980) Calcium transients in mammalian ventricular muscle. Eur Heart J 1 [Suppl A]: 5-15

Arunlakshana O, Schild HO (1959) Some quantitative uses of drug antagonists. Br J Pharmacol 14: 48-58

Bárány M, Bárány K (1981) Protein phosphorylation in cardiac and vascular smooth muscle. Am J Physiol 241: H117-H128

Barber R, Ray KP, Butcher RW (1980) Turnover of adenosine 3′,5′-monophosphate in WI-38 cultured fibroblasts. Biochemistry 19: 2560-2567

Benfey BG (1980) Cardiac α-adrenoceptors. Can J Physiol Pharmacol 58: 1145-1157

Berridge MJ (1981) Phosphatidylinositol hydrolysis: a multifunctional transducing mechanism. Mol Cell Endocrinol 24: 115-140

Berridge MJ (1984) Inositol trisphosphate and diacylglycerol as second messengers. Biochem J 220: 345-360

Berridge MJ, Irvine RF (1984) Inositol trisphosphate, a novel second messenger in cellular signal transduction. Nature 312: 315-321

Biegon RL, Epstein PM, Pappano AJ (1980) Muscarinic antagonism of the effects of a phosphodiesterase inhibitor (methylisobutylxanthine) in embryonic chick ventricle. J Pharmacol Exp Ther 215: 348-356

Blinks JR (1984) Methods for monitoring Ca^{++} concentrations with photoproteins in living cardiac cells. In: Dhalla NS (ed) Methods for studying heart membranes, vol 2. CRC Press, Boca Raton, pp 237-264

Blinks JR, Endoh M (1986) Modification of myofibrillar responsiveness to Ca^{++} as an inotropic mechanism. Circulation 73 [suppl] III-85-III-98

Blinks JR, Wier WG, Morgan JP, Hess P (1982) Regulation of intracellular [Ca^{2+}] by cardiotonic drugs. In: Yoshida H, Hagihara Y, Ebashi S (eds) Advances in pharmacology and therapeutics II, vol 3. Pergamon, Oxford, pp 205-216

Böhm M, Brückner R, Hackbarth I, Haubitz B, Linhart R, Meyer W, Schmidt B, Schmitz W, Scholz H (1984) Adenosine inhibition of catecholamine-induced increase in force of contraction in guinea-pig atrial and ventricular heart preparations: evidence against a cyclic AMP- and cyclic GMP-dependent effect. J Pharmacol Exp Ther 230: 483-492

Brodde OE, Motomura S, Endoh M, Schümann HJ (1978) Lack of correlation between the positive inotropic effect evoked by α-adrenoceptor stimulation and the levels of cyclic AMP and/or cyclic GMP in the isolated ventricle strip of the rabbit. J Mol Cell Cardiol 10: 207-219

Brodde OE, Inui J, Motomura S, Schümann HJ (1980) The mode of direct action of dopamine on the rabbit heart. J Cardiovasc Pharmacol 2: 567-582

Brown JH, Buxton IL, Brunton LL (1985) α_1-Adrenergic and muscarinic cholinergic stimulation of phosphoinositide hydrolysis in adult rat cardiomyocytes. Circ Res 57: 532-537

Brückner R, Scholz H (1984) Effects of α-adrenoceptor stimulation with phenylephrine in the presence of propranolol on force of contraction, slow inward current and cyclic AMP content in the bovine heart. Br J Pharmacol 82: 223-232

Brückner R, Meyer W, Mügge A, Schmitz W, Scholz H (1984) α-Adrenoceptor-mediated positive inotropic effect of phenylephrine in isolated human ventricular myocardium. Eur J Pharmacol 99: 345-347

Brückner R, Mügge A, Scholz H (1985) Existence and functional role of alpha$_1$-adrenoceptors in the mammalian heart. J Mol Cell Cardiol 17: 639-645

Ciaraldi T, Marinetti GV (1977) Thyroxine and propylthiouracil effects in vivo on alpha and beta adrenergic receptors in rat heart. Biochem Biophys Res Commun 74: 984-991

Cole HA, Perry SV (1975) The phosphorylation of troponin I from cardiac muscle. Biochem J 149: 525-533

Demaille JG, Pechère J-F (deceased) et al. (1983) The control of contractility by protein phosphorylation. Adv Cyclic Nucleotide Res 15: 337-371

Dumont JE, Miot F, Erneux C, Couchie D, Cochaux P, Gervy-Decoster C, Van Sande J, Wells JN (1984) Negative regulation of cyclic AMP levels by activation of cyclic nucleotide phosphodies-

terases: the example of the dog thyroid. Adv Cyclic Nucleotide Protein Phosphorylation Res 16: 325-336
Endoh M (1979) Correlation of cyclic AMP and cyclic GMP levels with changes in contractile force of dog ventricular myocardium during cholinergic antagonism of positive inotropic actions of histamine, glucagon, theophylline and papaverine. Jpn J Pharmacol 29: 855-864
Endoh M (1980) The time course of changes in cyclic nucleotide levels during cholinergic inhibition of positive inotropic actions of isoprenaline and theophylline in the isolated canine ventricular myocardium. Naunyn-Schmiedebergs Arch Pharmacol 312: 175-182
Endoh M (1982) Adrenoceptors and the myocardial inotropic response: do alpha and beta receptor sites functionally coexist? In: Kalsner S (ed) Trends in autonomic pharmacology, vol 2. Urban and Schwarzenberg, Baltimore, pp 303-322
Endoh M, Blinks JR (1984) Regulation of intracellular Ca^{++} transients and Ca^{++} sensitivity of myofibrils via α- and β-adrenoceptors in the rabbit papillary muscle. Cell Calcium 5: 301
Endoh M, Blinks JR (1986) Actions of sympathomimetic amines on the Ca^{++} transients and contractions of rabbit myocardium: comparison of effects mediated through alpha- and beta-adrenoceptors. Circ Res (submitted)
Endoh M, Motomura S (1979) Differentiation by cholinergic stimulation of positive inotropic actions mediated via α- and β-adrenoceptors in the rabbit heart. Life Sci 25: 759-768
Endoh M, Schümann HJ (1975a) Frequency-dependence of the positive inotropic effect of methoxamine and naphazoline mediated by α-adrenoceptors in the isolated rabbit papillary muscle. Naunyn-Schmiedebergs Arch Pharmacol 287: 377-389
Endoh M, Schümann HJ (1975b) Effects of papaverine on isolated rabbit papillary muscle. Eur J Pharmacol 30: 213-220
Endoh M, Yamashita S (1980) Adenosine antagonizes the positive inotropic action mediated via β-, but not α-adrenoceptors in the rabbit papillary muscle. Eur J Pharmacol 65: 445-448
Endoh M, Wagner J, Schümann HJ (1975) Influence of temperature on the positive inotropic effects mediated by α- and β-adrenoceptors in the isolated rabbit papillary muscle. Naunyn-Schmiedebergs Arch Pharmacol 287: 61-72
Endoh M, Brodde OE, Reinhardt D, Schümann HJ (1976a) Frequency dependence of cyclic AMP in mammalian myocardium. Nature 261: 716-717
Endoh M, Schümann HJ, Krappitz N, Hillen B (1976b) α-Adrenoceptors mediating positive inotropic effects on the ventricular myocardium: some aspects of structure-activity relationship of sympathomimetic amines. Jpn J Pharmacol 26: 179-190
Endoh M, Hillen B, Schümann HJ (1977) Influence of temperature and frequency on the positive inotropic action of phenylephrine in the isolated rabbit papillary muscle. Arch Int Pharmacodyn 228: 213-221
Endoh M, Shimizu T, Yanagisawa T (1978) Characterization of adrenoceptors mediating positive inotropic responses in the ventricular myocardium of the dog. Br J Pharmacol 64: 53-61
Endoh M, Satoh K, Taira N (1982) α-Adrenoceptors mediating the positive inotropic effect of phenylephrine in the right ventricular muscle of the monkey *(Macaca fuscata)*. Naunyn-Schmiedebergs Arch Pharmacol 318: 370-373
Endoh M, Maruyama M, Yanagisawa T (1984) Cholera toxin-induced changes in force of contraction and cyclic AMP levels in canine ventricular myocardium: inhibition by carbachol. Life Sci 35: 2397-2406
Endoh M, Maruyama M, Iijima T (1985) Attenuation of muscarinic cholinergic inhibition by islet-activating protein in the heart. Am J Physiol (Heart Circ) 249: H309-H320
Endoh M, Yanagisawa T, Taira N, Blinks JR (1986) Effects of new inotropic agents on cyclic nucleotide metabolism and calcium transients in canine ventricular muscle. Circulation 73 [suppl] III117-III133
England PJ (1975) Correlation between contraction and phosphorylation of the inhibitory subunit of troponin in perfused rat heart. FEBS Lett 50: 57-60
Fain JF, García-Sáinz JA (1980) Role of phosphatidylinositol turnover in $alpha_1$- and of adenylate cyclase inhibition in $alpha_2$-effects of catecholamines. Life Sci 26: 1183-1194
Glossman H, Hornung R (1980) Calcium- and potassium-channel blockers interact with α-adrenoceptors. Mol Cell Endocrinol 19: 243-251
Gross G, Lues I (1985) Thyroid-dependent alterations of myocardial adrenoceptors and adrenoceptor-mediated responses in the rat. Naunyn-Schmiedebergs Arch Pharmacol 329: 427-439

Guicheney P, Garay RP, Levy-Marchal C, Meyer P (1978) Biochemical evidence for presynaptic and postsynaptic α-adrenoceptors in rat heart membranes: positive homotropic cooperativity of presynaptic binding. Proc Natl Acad Sci USA 75: 6285-6289
Hashimoto H, Nakashima M (1978) Influence of thyroid hormone on the positive inotropic effects mediated by α- and β-adrenoceptors in isolated guinea pig atria and rabbit papillary muscles. Eur J Pharmacol 50: 337-347
Herzig JW, Köhler G, Pfitzer G, Rüegg JC, Wölffle G (1981) Cyclic AMP inhibits contractility of detergent treated glycerol extracted cardiac muscle. Pflügers Arch 391: 208-212
Hoh JFY, McGrath PA, Hale RT (1977) Electrophoretic analysis of multiple forms of rat cardiac myosin: effects of hypophysectomy and thyroxine replacement. J Mol Cell Cardiol 10: 1053-1076
Holroyde MJ, Howe E, Solaro RJ (1979) Modification of calcium requirements for activation of cardiac myofibrillar ATPase by cyclic AMP dependent phosphorylation. Biochem Biophys Acta 586: 63-69
Imai S (1961) The effects of methoxamine upon the membrane resting and action potentials of the guinea pig's ventricular muscle fibres. Jpn J Physiol 11: 54-61
Inui J, Brodde OE, Schümann HJ (1982) Influence of acetylcholine on the positive inotropic effect evoked by α- or β-adrenoceptor stimulation in the rabbit heart. Naunyn-Schmiedebergs Arch Pharmacol 320: 152-159
Iwasa T, Hosey M (1983) Cholinergic antagonism of β-adrenergic stimulation of cardiac membrane protein phosphorylation in situ. J Biol Chem 258: 4571-4575
Jakobs KH, Aktories K, Schultz G (1984) Mechanisms and components involved in adenylate cyclase inhibition by hormones. Adv Cyclic Nucleotide Res 17: 135-143
Karliner JS, Barnes P, Hamilton CA, Dollery CT (1979) α_1-Adrenergic receptors in guinea pig myocardium: identification by binding of a new radioligand, (^{3}H)-prazosin. Biochem Biophys Res Commun 90: 142-149
Karliner JS, Motulsky HJ, Dunlap J, Brown JH, Insel PA (1982) Verapamil competitively inhibits α_1-adrenergic and muscarinic but not β-adrenergic receptors in rat myocardium. J Cardiovasc Pharmacol 4: 515-520
Katz AM (1983) Cyclic adenosine monophosphate effects on the myocardium: a man who blows hot and cold with one breath. J Am Coll Cardiol 2: 143-149
Kaumann AJ, Blinks JR (1980) Stimulant and depressant effects of β-adrenoceptor blocking agents on isolated heart muscle: a possible inotropic effect not mediated through adrenoceptors. Naunyn-Schmiedebergs Arch Pharmacol 311: 205-218
Kunos G (1977) Thyroid hormone-dependent interconversion of myocardial α- and β-adrenoceptors in the rat. Br J Pharmacol 59: 177-189
Ledda F, Marchetti P, Mugelli A (1975) Studies on the positive inotropic effect of phenylephrine: a comparison with isoprenaline. Br J Pharmacol 54: 83-90
Ledda F, Mantelli L, Mugelli A (1980) α-Sympathomimetic amines and calcium-mediated action potentials in guinea-pig ventricular muscle. Br J Pharmacol 69: 565-571
Lefkowitz RJ, Stadel JM, Cerione RA, Strulovici B, Caron MG (1984) Structure and function of β-adrenergic receptors: regulation of the molecular level. Adv Cyclic Nucleotide Protein Phosphorylation Res 17: 19-28
Macleod KM (1985) The interaction of carbachol and forskolin in rabbit papillary muscles. Eur J Pharmacol 107: 95-99
Marban E, Rink TJ, Tsien RW, Tsien RY (1980) Free calcium in heart muscle at rest and during contraction measured with Ca^{2+}-sensitive microelectrodes. Nature 286: 845-850
Martin AF, Pagani D, Solaro RJ (1982) Thyroxine-induced redistribution of isozymes of rabbit ventricular myosin. Circ Res 50: 117-124
McClellan GB, Winegrad S (1978) The regulation of the calcium sensitivity of the contractile system in mammalian cardiac muscle. J Gen Physiol 72: 737-764
McConnaughey MM, Jones LR, Watanabe AM, Besch HR Jr, Williams LT, Lefkowitz RJ (1979) Thyroxine and propylthiouracil effects on alpha- and beta-adrenergic receptor number, ATPase activities, and sialic acid content of rat cardiac membrane vesicles. J Cardiovasc Pharmacol 1: 609-623
Meeker RB, Harden TK (1982) Muscarinic cholinergic receptor-mediated activation of phosphodiesterase. Mol Pharmacol 22: 310-319

Michell RH (1983) Polyphosphoinositide breakdown as the initiating reaction in receptor-stimulated inositol phospholipid metabolism. Life Sci 32: 2083-2085

Miura Y, Inui J, Imamura H (1978) Alpha-adrenoceptor-mediated restoration of calcium-dependent potential in the partially depolarized rabbit papillary muscle. Naunyn-Schmiedebergs Arch Pharmacol 301: 201-205

Mope L, McClellan GB, Winegrad S (1980) Calcium sensitivity of the contractile system and phosphorylation of troponin in hyperpermeable cardiac cells. J Gen Physiol 75: 271-282

Morgan JP, Blinks JR (1982) Intracellular Ca^{2+} transient in the cat papillary muscle. Can J Physiol Pharmacol 60: 524-528

Morgan JP, Morgan KG (1984) Calcium and cardiovascular function: intracellular calcium levels during contraction and relaxation of mammalian cardiac and vascular smooth muscle as detected with aequorin. Am J Med 77 (5 A): 33-46

Motulsky HJ, Snavely MD, Hughes RJ, Insel PA (1983) Interaction of verapamil and other calcium channel blockers with α_1- and α_2-adrenergic receptors. Circ Res 52: 226-231

Movsesian MA, Nishikawa M, Adelstein RS (1984) Phosphorylation of phospholamban by calcium-activated, phospholipid-dependent protein kinase: stimulation of cardiac sarcoplasmic reticulum calcium uptake. J Biol Chem 259: 8029-8032

Mukherjee A, Haghani Z, Brady J, Bush L, McBride W, Buja LM, Willerson JT (1983) Differences in myocardial α- and β-adrenergic receptor numbers in different species. Am J Physiol 245: H957-H961

Murad F, Chi YM, Rall TW, Sutherland EW (1962) Adenyl cyclase: III. the effect of catecholamines and choline esters on the formation of adenosine 3′,5′-phosphate by preparations from cardiac muscle and liver. J Biol Chem 237: 1233-1238

Nakashima M, Maeda K, Sekiya A, Hagino Y (1971) Effect of hypothyroid status on myocardial responses to sympathomimetic drugs. Jpn J Pharmacol 21: 819-825

Nakashima M, Tsuru H, Shigei T (1973) Stimulant action of methoxamine in the isolated atria of normal and 6-propyl-2-thiouracil-fed rats. Jpn J Pharmacol 23: 307-312

Nayler WG (1972) Comparative partial agonist activity of β-adrenoceptor antagonists. Br J Pharmacol 45: 382-384

Nishizuka Y (1983) Phospholipid degradation and signal translation for protein phosphorylation. Trends Biochem Sci 8: 13-16

Osnes JB, Refsum H, Skomedal T, Øye I (1978) Qualitative differences between β-adrenergic and α-adrenergic inotropic effects in rat heart muscle. Acta Pharmacol Toxicol 42: 235-247

Pappano AJ, Hartigan PM, Coutu MD (1982) Acetylcholine inhibits positive inotropic effect of cholera toxin in ventricular muscle. Am J Physiol 243: H434-H441

Ray KP, England PJ (1976) Phosphorylation of the inhibitory subunit of troponin and its effect on the calcium dependence of cardiac myofibril adenosine triphosphatase. FEBS Lett 70: 11-16

Sanchez-Chapula J (1981) Multiple effects of putative α-adrenoceptor agonists on the electrical and mechanical activity of guinea-pig papillary muscle. Naunyn-Schmiedebergs Arch Pharmacol 316: 108-111

Scholz H (1980) Effects of beta- and alpha-adrenoceptor activators and adrenergic transmitter releasing agents on the mechanical activity of the heart. In: Szekeres L (ed) Adrenergic activators and inhibitors. Springer, Berlin Heidelberg New York, pp 651-733

Schümann HJ (1980) Are there α-adrenoceptors in the mammalian heart? Trends Pharmacol Sci 1: 195-197

Schümann HJ, Brodde OE (1979) Demonstration of α-adrenoceptors in the rabbit heart by [^{3}H]-dihydroergocryptine binding. Naunyn-Schmiedebergs Arch Pharmacol 308: 191-198

Schümann HJ, Endoh M (1976) α-Adrenoceptors in the ventricular myocardium: clonidine, naphazoline and methoxamine as partial α-agonists exerting a competitive dualism in action to phenylephrine. Eur J Pharmacol 36: 413-421

Schümann HJ, Endoh M, Wagner J (1974) Positive inotropic effects of phenylephrine in the isolated rabbit papillary muscle mediated both by α- and β-adrenoceptors. Naunyn-Schmiedebergs Arch Pharmacol 284: 133-148

Schümann HJ, Endoh M, Brodde OE (1975) The time course of the effects of β- and α-adrenoceptor stimulation by isoprenaline and methoxamine on the contractile force and cAMP level of the isolated rabbit papillary muscle. Naunyn-Schmiedebergs Arch Pharmacol 289: 291-302

Schümann HJ, Motomura S, Endoh M, Brodde OE (1977) Comparison of the mechanisms under-

lying the positive inotropic actions of dopamine, adrenaline and isoprenaline on the isolated rabbit papillary muscle. Naunyn-Schmiedebergs Arch Pharmacol 297: 257-267
Schümann HJ, Wagner J, Knorr A, Reidemeister JChr, Sadony V, Schramm G (1978) Demonstration in human atrial preparations of α-adrenoceptors mediating positive inotropic effects. Naunyn-Schmiedebergs Arch Pharmacol 302: 333-336
Sekar MC, Roufogalis BD (1984) Comparison of muscarinic and alpha-adrenergic receptors in rat atria based on phosphoinositide turnover. Life Sci 35: 1527-1533
Sharma VK, Banerjee SP (1978) α-Adrenergic receptor in rat heart: effects of thyroidectomy. J Biol Chem 253: 5277-5279
Shibata S, Seriguchi DG, Iwadare S, Ishida Y, Shibata T (1980) The regional and species differences of the activation of myocardial alpha-adrenoceptors by phenylephrine and methoxamine. Gen Pharmacol 11: 173-180
Skomedal T, Aass H, Osnes JB (1984) Specific binding of (^{3}H) prazosin to myocardial cells isolated from adult rats. Biochem Pharmacol 33: 1897-1906
Smigel M, Katada T, Northup JK, Bokoch GM, Ui M, Gilman AG (1984) Mechanisms of guanine nucleotide-mediated regulation of adenylate cyclase activity. Adv Cyclic Nucleotide Protein Phosphorylation Res 17: 1-18
Solaro RJ (1982) The role of calcium in the contraction of the heart. In: Flaim SF, Zelis R (eds) Calcium blockers: mechanisms of action and clinical applications. Urban and Schwarzenberg, Baltimore, pp 21-36
Spiegel AM, Gierschik P, Levine MA, Downs RW (1985) Clinical implications of guanine nucleotide-binding proteins as receptor-effector couplers. N Engl J Med 312: 26-33
Stull JT (1980) Phosphorylation of contractile proteins in relation to muscle function. Adv Cyclic Nucleotide Res 13: 39-93
Sutherland EW, Robison GA, Butcher RW (1968) Some aspects of the biological role of adenosine 3′,5′-monophosphate (cyclic AMP). Circulation 37: 279-306
Tada M, Katz AM (1982) Phosphorylation of the sarcoplasmic reticulum and sarcolemma. Ann Rev Physiol 44: 401-423
Tada M, Kirchberger MA, Iorio JAM, Katz AM (1975) Control of cardiac sarcolemmal adenylate cyclase and sodium, potassium-activated adenosinetriphosphatase activities. Circ Res 36: 8-17
Takai Y, Kishimoto A, Kawahara Y, Minakuchi R, Sano K, Kikkawa U, Mori T, Yu B, Kaibuchi K, Nishizuka Y (1981) Calcium and phosphatidylinositol turnover as signalling for transmembrane control of protein phosphorylation. Adv Cyclic Nucleotide Res 14: 301-313
Tsai JS, Chen A (1978) Effect of *L*-triiodothyronine on (–)^{3}H-dihydroalprenolol binding and cyclic AMP response to (–)adrenaline in cultured heart cells. Nature 275: 138-140
Tsien RW (1977) Cyclic AMP and contractile activity in heart. Adv Cyclic Nucleotide Res 8: 368-420
Uchida T, Bhatnagar GM, Lakatta EG, Filburn CR (1982) Alpha-adrenergic stimulation of $^{32}PO_4$ labelling of phosphatidylinositol (PI) and phosphatidic acid (PA) in cultured rat heart cells. Fed Proc 41: 1523
Ui M (1984) Islet-activating protein, pertussis toxin: a probe for functions of the inhibitory guanine nucleotide regulatory component of adenylate cyclase. Trends Pharmacol Sci 5: 277-279
Ui M, Katada T, Maruyama T, Kurose H, Yajima M, Tamura M, Nakamura T, Nogimori K (1984) Iselet-activating protein, pertussis toxin: a specific uncoupler of receptor-mediated inhibition of adenylate cyclase. Adv Cyclic Nucleotide Protein Phosphorylation Res 17: 145-151
Van Sande J, Erneux C, Dumont JE (1977) Negative control of TSH action by iodide and acetylcholine: mechanism of action in intact thyroid cells. J Cyclic Nucleotide Res 3: 335-345
Wagner J, Brodde OE (1978) On the presence and distribution of α-adrenoceptors in the heart of various mammalian species. Naunyn-Schmiedebergs Arch Pharmacol 302: 239-254
Wagner J, Schümann HJ, Knorr A, Rohm N, Reidemeister JChr (1980) Stimulation by adrenaline and dopamine but not by noradrenaline of myocardial α-adrenoceptors mediating positive inotropic effects in human atrial preparations. Naunyn-Schmiedebergs Arch Pharmacol 312: 99-102
Watanabe AM, Besch HR Jr (1975) Interaction between cyclic adenosine monophosphate and cyclic guanosine monophosphate in guinea pig ventricular myocardium. Circ Res 37: 309-317
Williams LT, Lefkowitz RJ, Watanabe AM, Hathaway DR, Besch HR Jr (1977) Thyroid hormone regulation of β-adrenergic receptor number. J Biol Chem 252: 2787-2789

Williams RS, Lefkowitz RJ (1978) Alpha-adrenergic receptors in rat myocardium: identification by binding of [^{3}H] dihydroergocryptine. Circ Res 43: 721-727
Williams RS, Lefkowitz RJ (1979) Thyroid hormone regulation of alpha-adrenergic receptors: studies in rat myocardium. J Cardiovasc Pharmacol 1: 181-189
Winegrad S (1984) Regulation of cardiac contractile proteins: correlations between physiology and biochemistry. Circ Res 55: 565-574
Winegrad S, McClellan G, Tucker M, Lin LE (1983) Cyclic AMP regulation of myosin isozymes in mammalian cardiac muscle. J Gen Physiol 81: 749-765
Yamamoto K, Ohtsuki I (1982) Effect of phosphorylation of porcine cardiac troponin I by 3′:5′-cyclic AMP-dependent protein kinase on the actomyosin ATPase activity. J Biochem 91: 1669-1677
Yamashita S, Endoh M (1981) Adrenoceptors mediating the positive inotropic effect in the canine atrial myocardium. Jpn J Pharmacol 31: 649-651

The Functional Role of the Coexistence of β_1- and β_2-Adrenoceptors in the Human Heart

O.-E. Brodde

Abteilung für Nieren- und Hochdruckkranke, Nephrologisches Labor, Medizinische Klinik und Poliklinik, Universitätsklinikum Essen, Hufelandstraße 55, 4300 Essen 1, Federal Republic of Germany

Introduction

The subclassification of β-adrenoceptors into the subtypes β_1 and β_2 was originally postulated by Lands et al. (1967 a, b), based on the findings that sympathomimetic agents evoked their effects on different tissues with different orders of potency. β_1- and β_2-Adrenoceptors differ in their relative affinities for the endogenous catecholamines noradrenaline and adrenaline. At β_1-adrenoceptors, which mediate cardiac effects and lipolysis, noradrenaline and adrenaline are equipotent; on the other hand, at β_2-adrenoceptors, which mediate smooth muscle relaxation, adrenaline is approximately 10–30 times more potent than noradrenaline. During the past few years, growing evidence has accumulated that β_1- and β_2-adrenoceptors are not always organ-specifically distributed, but that both β-adrenoceptor subtypes can coexist in a single organ (for recent reviews, see Minneman et al. 1981; Stiles et al. 1984). This was first suggested in 1972 by Carlsson et al., who showed that equal submaximal chronotropic responses of the cat heart to β-adrenergic agonists were antagonized to a different extent by practolol (a β_1-selective antagonist) and H 35/25 (a β_2-selective antagonist). Subsequently, similar effects have been obtained in several in vivo and in vitro experiments in cat, dog and guinea pig hearts as well as in guinea pig and rabbit trachea (for references, see Daly and Levy 1979), thus supporting the concept of the coexistence of β_1- and β_2-adrenoceptors in a single organ.

Radioligand binding studies have enabled for the first time the *direct* determination of the tissue concentration of β-adrenoceptors and thus the responsiveness of the tissues to β-adrenergic stimulation (Lefkowitz 1978; Hoffman and Lefkowitz 1980). With the use of this technique, it is also possible to determine the relative proportion of β_1- and β_2-adrenoceptors present in a tissue. The technique most widely used in order to quantify the relative amount of β_1- and β_2-adrenoceptors is the assessment of inhibition of binding of unselective β-adrenoceptor radioligands such as (−)-[^{3}H]dihydroalprenolol, (±)-[^{125}I]iodohydroxybenzylpindolol or (±)-[^{125}I]iodocyanopindolol *(ICYP)* by unlabelled drugs that have shown in vitro selectivity for β_1- or β_2-adrenoceptors. From the resulting competition curves, the relative proportion of β_1- and β_2-adrenoceptors can be calculated using various analytical methods (Minneman et al. 1979; Molinoff et al. 1981; DeLean et al. 1982). With the use of this technique, the coexistence of β_1- and β_2-adrenoceptors has been demonstrated in the heart of rat, guinea pig, cat and rabbit as well as in the lung of rat, rabbit and guinea pig (for recent reviews, see Minneman et al. 1981; Stiles et al. 1984). However, little is known about the properties of β-adrenoceptors in the hu-

New Aspects of the Role of Adrenoceptors in the
Cardiovascular System/Ed. by Grobecker et al.

man heart. In the present study, therefore, the β-adrenoceptor subtypes present in human right atrial appendages were identified by the use of ICYP binding. In addition, the question of which β-adrenoceptor subtype is involved in activation of adenylate cyclase in the human right atrium was studied. Finally, the β-adrenoceptor subtype mediating the positive inotropic effects of isoprenaline and of the selective β_2-agonist procaterol (Yoshizaki et al. 1976; Yabuuchi 1977) was characterized on the isolated, electrically driven muscle strip of the human right atrial appendage. For this study, the highly selective β_1-antagonist bisoprolol (Schliep and Harting 1984; Wang et al. 1985) and the highly selective β_2-antagonist ICI 118,551 (Bilski et al. 1983) were used.

Subjects and Methods

Human right atrial appendages were obtained from 35 patients (aged 9-71 years; mean age, 48.7 ± 7.4 years) undergoing elective coronary artery bypass grafting. No patient suffered from acute myocardial failure, and none of the patients had been treated with catecholamines during the 3 weeks before surgery. Premedication consisted of flunitrazepam and atropine, and the operation was performed under balanced anaesthesia using fentanyl and isoflurane or etomidate and flunitrazepam. In some cases, N_2O was added. Pancuronium was used as a muscle relaxant. In all patients, the right atrial appendages were removed under normothermic conditions before cardiopulmonary bypass. Immediately after removal, all specimens were placed in a sealed vial with Krebs-Henseleit solution (composition, see below) aerated by carbogen (95% O_2, 5% CO_2) at room temperature and transported immediately to the laboratory. The preparation of the tissues began within 5-15 min after surgical removal. For the physiological experiments, the atrial appendages were dissected to yield trabecular strips (diameter 1 mm or less) 4-5 mm in length without endocardial damage. The preparation was performed in oxygenated Krebs-Henseleit solution at room temperature in order to minimize inadequate oxygenation. The dissection was carried out to obtain strips in which the fibres ran parallel to the length. Only tissues which could be divided into at least four strips were used. The preparations were mounted in a 50-ml organ bath containing Krebs-Henseleit solution with the following composition (mmol/liter): NaCl 119; $CaCl_2$ 2.5; KCl 4.8; $MgSO_4$ 1.2; KH_2PO_4 1.2; $NaHCO_3$ 24.9; glucose 10.0; ascorbic acid 0.057. The prepared tissues were equilibrated with carbogen at a temperature of 37 °C, were electrically stimulated by square wave impulses of 5-ms duration and a voltage 20% above threshold at a frequency of stimulation of 1 Hz. The developed tension of the atria maintained under a resting tension of 4.9 mN was recorded via a strain gauge on a Hellige recorder. All preparations were incubated for 2 h with 5 μmol/liter phenoxybenzamine to avoid tissue uptake of isoprenaline. Cumulative dose-response curves for the positive inotropic effects of isoprenaline and procaterol were determined as recently described (Zerkowski et al. 1986). The procedure used for preparation of human right atrial membranes for characterization of the β-adrenoceptors by ICYP binding and for assessment of adenylate cyclase activity essentially followed that which was recently described by Brodde et al. (1983, 1984).

Statistical Evaluations

The experimental data given in the text, as well as in the figures and tables included in this paper are means ± SEM of *n* experiments. The equilibrium dissociation constants (K_D) and the maximal number of binding sites (B_{max}) were calculated from plots according to the method of Scatchard (1949). Analysis of inhibition of ICYP binding by β_1- and β_2-selective drugs was performed by nonlinear regression analysis under the assumption of two independent binding sites, as described by Engel et al. (1981). K_I values for inhibition of isoprenaline-stimulated adenylate cyclase activity by propranolol were determined according to the equation of Cheng and Prusoff (1973):

$$K_I = \frac{IC_{50}}{\frac{S}{K_D} + 1}$$

where IC_{50} is the concentration of propranolol necessary to inhibit isoprenaline stimulation by 50%, *S* is the concentration of isoprenaline (10 μmol/liter) in the assay and $K_D = K_{act}$ for stimulation of adenylate cyclase by isoprenaline. K_{act} values were determined as the concentration necessary to produce 50% for maximal stimulation of adenylate cyclase activity.

pD_2 Values (i.e. the negative logarithm of the molar concentration of agonists causing half-maximal effects) were determined as described by Van Rossum (1963). pA_2 Values (i.e. the negative logarithm of the molar concentration of bisoprolol and ICI 118,551 which produces a twofold shift to the right of the dose-response curve for procaterol) were determined according to Arunlakshana and Schild (1959).

Results

Demonstration of β_1- and β_2-Adrenoceptors in Membranes from Human Right Atrium

To determine the density of β-adrenoceptors in membranes derived from human right atrial appendages, concentration-dependent binding of the highly selective β-adrenoceptor antagonist radioligand ICYP was studied. Binding of ICYP was saturable and of high affinity; Fig. 1 shows a typical experiment. Scatchard analysis (1949) of the binding data (Fig. 1 inset) resulted in a single line, suggesting that ICYP labels only *one* class of binding sites. From the Scatchard plot, a maximal number of binding sites of 86.4 ± 7.4 fmol ICYP specifically bound per mg protein was obtained; the K_D value for ICYP was 53 ± 6 pmol/liter ($n = 4$).

To characterize the β-adrenoceptor subtypes present in human right atrium, inhibition of ICYP binding by several β-adrenergic drugs was investigated. β-Adrenergic agonists inhibited ICYP binding with an order of potency of isoprenaline > adrenaline = noradrenaline (Fig. 2), which is typical for β_1-adrenoceptors (Lands et al. 1967 a, b). Binding was stereospecific, as indicated by the 100-fold greater potency of (–)-propranolol than its (+)-isomer in inhibiting binding (Fig. 2). Inhibition of

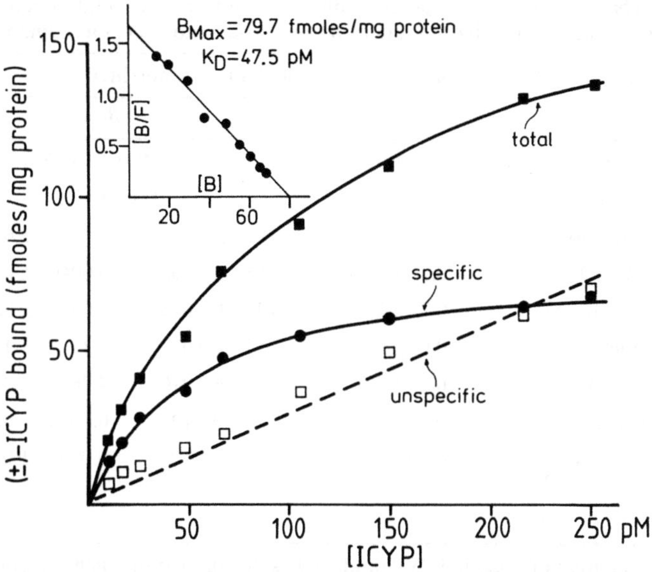

Fig. 1. Binding of ICYP to membranes from human right atria as function of increasing ICYP concentrations. Binding was carried out at nine concentrations of ICYP ranging from 10 to 250 pmol/liter in the absence (■——■) and presence (□ - - - □) of 1 μmol/liter (–)-propranolol to determine specific binding (●——●). *Ordinate,* ICYP bound (fmol/mg protein); *abscissa,* free ICYP concentration (pmol/liter). *Inset,* Scatchard plot of specific ICYP binding. The figure shows a typical saturation experiment. From Brodde et al. (1983)

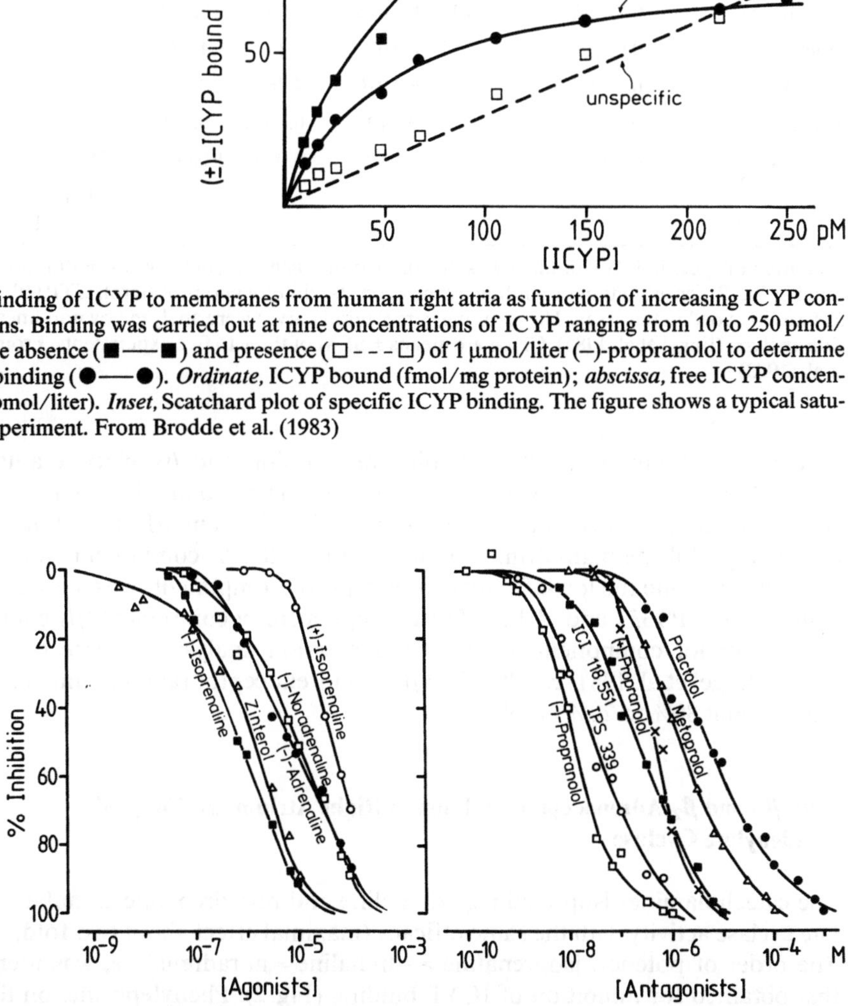

Fig. 2. Inhibition of specific ICYP binding to membranes from human right atria by β-adrenergic agonists and antagonists. Membranes were incubated with ICYP (40000–60000 cpm; 40–60 pmol/liter) in the presence or absence of 9–14 concentrations of the indicated agents, and specific binding was determined. For inhibition of binding by agonists, GTP (10^{-4} mol/liter) was included in the assay. "100%" inhibition refers to inhibition of specific binding by 1 μmol/liter (–)-propranolol. Each value is the mean of three experiments with a SEM of less than 4%. From Brodde et al. (1983)

Table 1. K_I Values and pseudo-Hill coefficients (n_H) for inhibition of ICYP binding by β-adrenergic drugs and relative amount of β_1- and β_2-adrenoceptors in human right atrial appendage

Drugs	n_H	K_I Values (μmol/liter)		Receptor subtypes β_1/β_2 (%)
		β_1	β_2	
(−)-Propranolol	0.99 ± 0.11	0.007 ± 0.003		
(+)-Propranolol		0.66 ± 0.05		
Betaxolol	0.69 ± 0.06	0.027 ± 0.002	1.9 ± 0.09	82/18
IPS 339	0.76 ± 0.05	0.084 ± 0.008	0.0046 ± 0.0003	86/14
ICI 118,551	0.72 ± 0.07	0.17 ± 0.016	0.00095 ± 0.0001	87/13
Practolol	0.62 ± 0.05	0.92 ± 0.07	15.3 ± 1.07	79/21
Metoprolol	0.77 ± 0.07	0.11 ± 0.010	4.76 ± 0.55	82/18
Zinterol	0.61 ± 0.08	0.92 ± 0.12	0.0090 ± 0.0014	83/17
Procaterol	0.70 ± 0.06	11.9 ± 1.52	0.099 ± 0.0042	76/24
				Mean, 82.1 ± 1.5/ 17.9 ± 1.5

Inhibition of specific ICYP binding was determined for each drug at 9–14 concentrations, as indicated in Fig. 2; for inhibition of binding by the agonists, zinterol and procaterol, GTP (10^{-4} mol/liter) was included in the assay. The resulting competition curves were analyzed by non-linear regression analysis (Engel et al. 1981). Given are means ± SEM of three to five experiments. From Brodde et al. (1983)

specific ICYP binding by β_1-(practolol, metoprolol) and β_2-selective antagonists (ICI 118,551, IPS339), however, resulted in biphasic competition curves (Fig. 2), suggesting the existence of two binding sites with different affinities. For practolol and metoprolol the high-affinity component (i.e. the β_1-component) was a major component, while the low-affinity component (β_2-component) was a minor one. In contrast, for IPS339 and ICI 118,551 the high-affinity component (β_2-component) was the minor component. Non-linear regression analysis of these competition curves (Engel et al. 1981) resulted in a β_1/β_2-adrenoceptor ratio in human right atrium of about 80% to 20% (Table 1).

Both β_1- and β_2-Adrenoceptors in Human Right Atrium are Coupled to Adenylate Cyclase

The catecholamines isoprenaline, adrenaline and noradrenaline stimulated adenylate cyclase activity with the same efficacy (maximal effect about two-fold, Fig. 3 A). The order of potency, isoprenaline > adrenaline = noradrenaline, was identical to that obtained for inhibition of ICYP binding (Fig. 2). Phenylephrine, on the other hand, stimulated adenylate cyclase activity only at high concentrations (> 10^{-5} mol/liter); its maximal effect was approximately 55% of that of isoprenaline. The (−)-isoprenaline-induced (10 μmol/liter) increase in adenylate cyclase activity was inhibited in a concentration-dependent and stereospecific manner by propranolol with the (−)-isomer being about 100 times more potent than the (+)-isomer

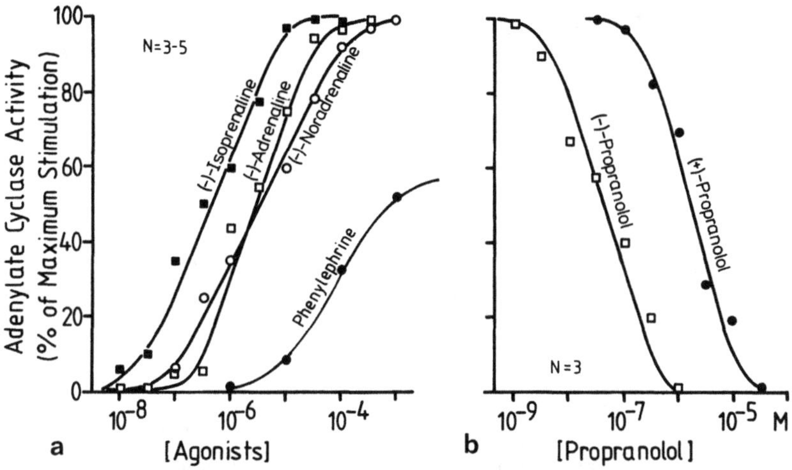

Fig. 3. **a** Effects of (—)-isoprenaline, (—)-adrenaline, (—)-noradrenaline and phenylephrine on adenylate cyclase activity in membranes from human right atria. *Ordinate,* percentage adenylate cyclase activity, where maximal stimulation is 100%. Basal activity was 7.7 ± 1.3 pmol cyclic AMP formed/min per mg protein (n = 12); isoprenaline, adrenaline and noradrenaline showed equal efficacy, i.e. activated adenylate cyclase to the same extent (about twofold). *Abscissa,* molar concentrations of agonists. **b** Inhibition of (—)-isoprenaline-stimulated adenylate cyclase activity (10 μmol/liter) in membranes from human right atria by (—)- and (+)-propranolol. *Ordinate,* adenylate cyclase activity as percentage of maximal stimulation by (—)-isoprenaline (basal activity: 8.2 ± 0.9 pmol cyclic AMP formed/min per mg protein (n = 6); (—)-isoprenaline-stimulated activity: 16.9 ± 1.8 pmol cyclic AMP formed/min per mg protein (n = 6)). *Abscissa,* molar concentrations of propranolol. Each value is the mean of three experiments with a SEM of less than 10%. From Brodde et al. (1983, 1984)

(Fig. 3 B). The K_I value of (—)-propranolol for inhibiting isoprenaline stimulated adenylate cyclase (3 nmol/liter) corresponded well to that obtained for inhibition of ICYP binding (7 nmol/liter, Table 1).

In addition to catecholamines, the β_2-selective agonists fenoterol and procaterol caused concentration-dependent increases in adenylate cyclase activity. The maximal effect, however, was only 43% and 64% respectively of that of isoprenaline (Fig. 4). The stimulation of the adenylate cyclase activity evoked by these compounds was not additive to the stimulation caused by isoprenaline, thus indicating that fenoterol and procaterol activate adenylate cyclase through β-adrenoceptor stimulation. The K_{act} values for fenoterol and procaterol (concentration necessary to cause 50% of maximal stimulation of adenylate cyclase) corresponded well to their K_I values for inhibition of ICYP binding to β_2-adrenoceptors in human right atrium (Table 2). The highly selective β_2-adrenoceptor antagonist ICI 118,551 inhibited procaterol-stimulated adenylate cyclase activity much more potently than it inhibited isoprenaline-stimulated activity (Fig. 5), while the β_1-selective antagonist betaxolol was more potent in inhibiting isoprenaline-stimulated activity. These results indicate that isoprenaline activates adenylate cyclase in human right atrium by β_1-adrenoceptor stimulation, whereas procaterol stimulates adenylate cyclase predominantly via β_2-adrenoceptors.

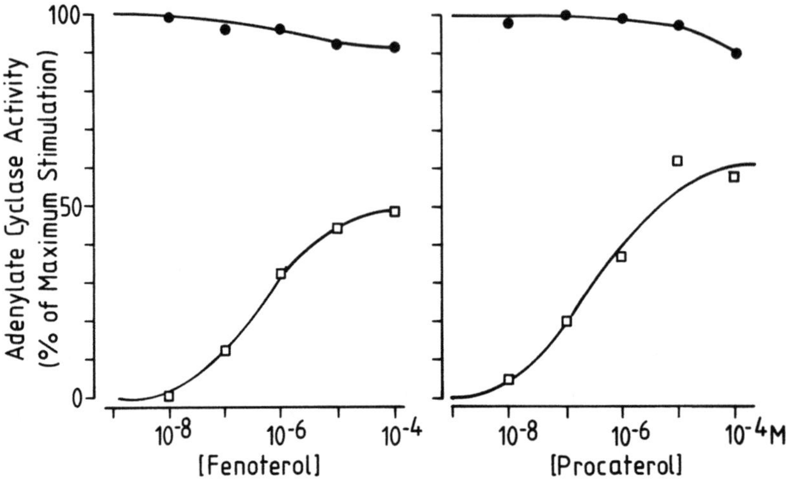

Fig. 4. Effects of fenoterol and procaterol on basal (□——□) or 10 µmol/liter isoprenaline stimulated (●——●) adenylate cyclase activity in membranes from human atria. Membranes were incubated under standard assay conditions in the absence or presence of 10 µmol/liter (–)-isoprenaline with different concentrations of fenoterol and procaterol ranging from 10^{-8}–10^{-4} mol/liter, and cyclic AMP formed was determined. *Ordinate,* percentage of adenylate cyclase activity, where maximal stimulation evoked by 10 µmol/liter (–)-isoprenaline is 100%; *abscissa,* molar concentrations of fenoterol and procaterol. Each value is the mean of four experiments with a SEM of less than 10%. From Brodde et al. (1984)

Table 2. K_{act} values for activation of adenylate cyclase activity in human right atrium by β-adrenergic agonists

	K_{act} values (µmol/liter)	Intrinsic activity	K_I values for inhibition of ICYP binding to human right atria (µmol/liter)	
			β_1-Adrenoceptors	β_2-Adrenoceptors
(–)-Isoprenaline	0.53 ± 0.05 (7)	1.0	0.42 ± 0.02 (5)	
(–)-Adrenaline	3.11 ± 0.21 (3)	1.0 ± 0.09 (3)	4.91 ± 0.52 (3)	
(–)-Noradrenaline	4.23 ± 0.31 (3)	1.0 ± 0.11 (3)	5.13 ± 0.44 (3)	
Phenylephrine	72.4 ± 9.8 (4)	0.53 ± 0.04 (4)	–	–
Procaterol	0.21 ± 0.03 (4)	0.64 ± 0.07 (4)	11.90 ± 1.52 (3)	0.099 ± 0.004 (3)
Fenoterol	0.66 ± 0.09 (4)	0.43 ± 0.04 (4)	2.21 ± 0.30 (4)	0.78 ± 0.11 (4)
Salbutamol	ND	0	–	–

ND, not determinable, since no activation up to 100 µmol/liter was observed; –, not determined
Given are means ± SEM; number of experiments in parentheses

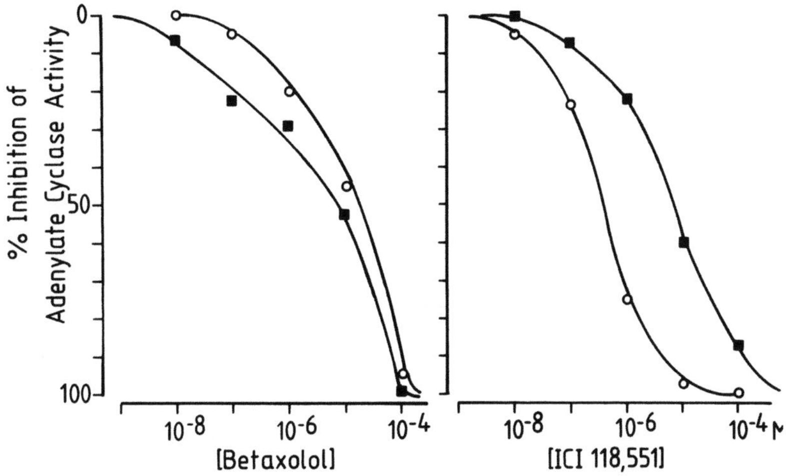

Fig. 5. Effects of betaxolol or ICI 118,551 on isoprenaline- or procaterol-stimulated adenylate cyclase activity in membranes from human right atria. Membranes were incubated under standard assay conditions with 10 µmol/liter (–)-isoprenaline (■——■) or 10 µmol/liter procaterol (O——O) in the absence or presence of different concentrations of betaxalol or ICI 118,551 ranging from 10^{-8} to 10^{-4} mol/liter and cyclic AMP formed was determined. *Ordinate*, percentage of inhibition of maximal stimulation of adenylate cyclase activity evoked by 10 µmol/liter (–)-isoprenaline *or* 10 µmol/liter procaterol; *abscissa*, molar concentrations of betaxolol and ICI 118,551. Given are means of three experiments with a SEM less than 10%. From Brodde et al. (1984)

Both β_1- and β_2-Adrenoceptors Are Involved in the Positive Inotropic Effects of β-Agonists on the Isolated Electrically Driven Human Right Atrium

The question of whether human atrial β_2-adrenoceptors are involved in the mechanical responses to β-agonists on the isolated electrically driven muscle strip of the human right atrial appendage was also investigated. To do this, the β-adrenoceptor subtypes mediating the positive inotropic effects of isoprenaline and of the selective β_2-agonist procaterol (Yoshizaki et al. 1976; Yabuuchi 1977) were characterized using the highly selective β_1-antagonist bisoprolol (Schliep and Harting 1984; Wang et al. 1985) and the highly selective β_2-antagonist ICI 118,551 (Bilski et al. 1983). Isoprenaline (10^{-9}–10^{-6} mol/liter; Fig. 6) and procaterol (10^{-9}–10^{-6} mol/liter; Fig. 7) induced concentration-dependent increases in force of contraction. In saturating concentrations (10^{-6} mol/liter isoprenaline; 3×10^{-7} mol/liter procaterol), both agonists produced the same maximum of the developed tension (isoprenaline: 7.93 ± 0.99 mN, $n=8$; procaterol: 7.25 ± 1.12 mN, $n=9$). The pD_2 value for isoprenaline was 7.73 ± 0.12 ($n=8$), and for procaterol it amounted to 8.03 ± 0.18 ($n=9$). ICI 118,551 (10^{-9}–10^{-7} mol/liter) and bisoprolol (10^{-9}–10^{-7} mol/liter) were nearly equipotent in antagonizing the positive inotropic effect of isoprenaline (Fig. 6). However, the slopes of the Schild plots for both antagonists against isoprenaline produced-inotropic effects were significantly less than 1.0 (bisoprolol: 0.61 ± 0.06, $n=4$; ICI 118,551: 0.48 ± 0.05, $n=4$) indicating interaction with β_1- and β_2-adrenoceptors.

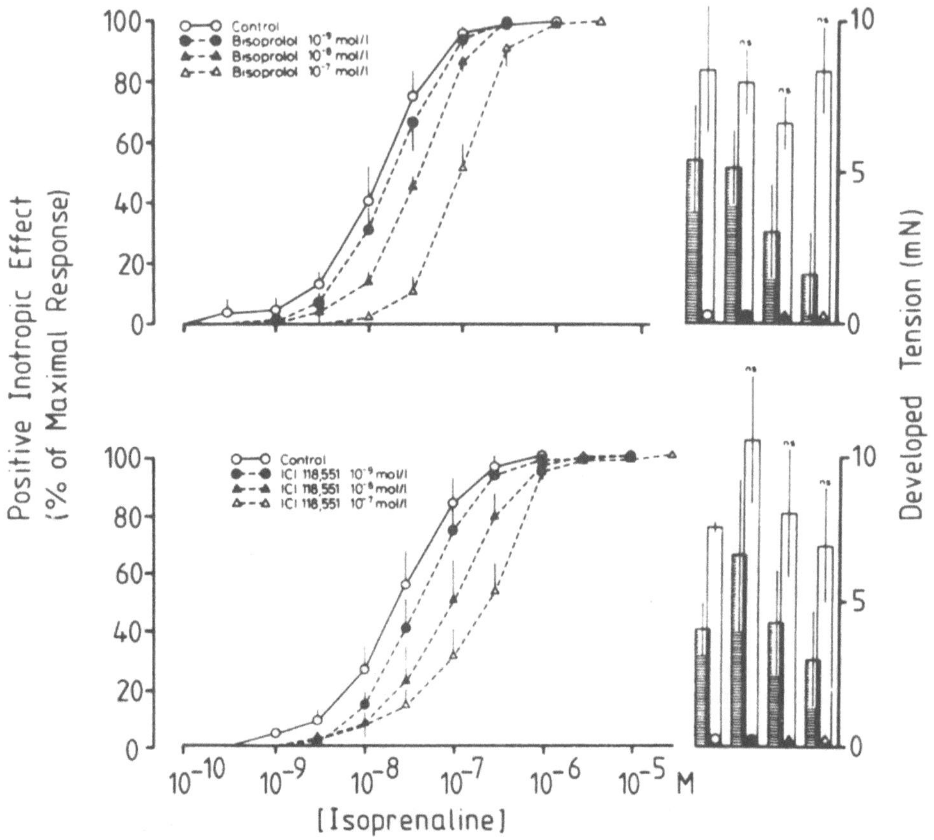

Fig. 6. Influence of bisoprolol and ICI 118,551 on the positive inotropic effect of isoprenaline on isolated muscle strips of human right atrial appendages. *Left ordinates,* positive inotropic effect as percentage of maximal response; *right ordinates,* basal (▤) and maximal developed tension (□) in the absence and presence of bisoprolol and ICI 118,551 respectively in mN. *Abscissa,* molar concentrations of isoprenaline. Given are means ± SEM of four experiments each. From Zerkowski et al. (1986)

On the other hand, ICI 118,551 (10^{-10}–10^{-8} mol/liter) was approximately 100 times more potent than bisoprolol (10^{-8}–10^{-6} mol/liter) in antagonizing the positive inotropic effect of the highly selective β_2-agonist procaterol (Fig. 7). In addition, the slopes of the Schild plots for antagonism of ICI 118,551 and bisoprolol against procaterol were not significantly different from unity (ICI 118,551: 0.87 ± 0.07, $n=6$; bisoprolol: 0.93 ± 0.08, $n=3$), indicating interaction with a homogeneous class of β-adrenoceptors. The pA_2 value of ICI 118,551 was 9.49 ± 0.06 ($n=3$), while for bisoprolol it amounted to 6.99 ± 0.03 ($n=3$).

Distribution of β_1- and β_2-Adrenoceptors in Different Parts of the Human Heart

Finally, we investigated the regional distribution of β_1- and β_2-adrenoceptors in the human heart. For this purpose, we analyzed competition curves of the highly selec-

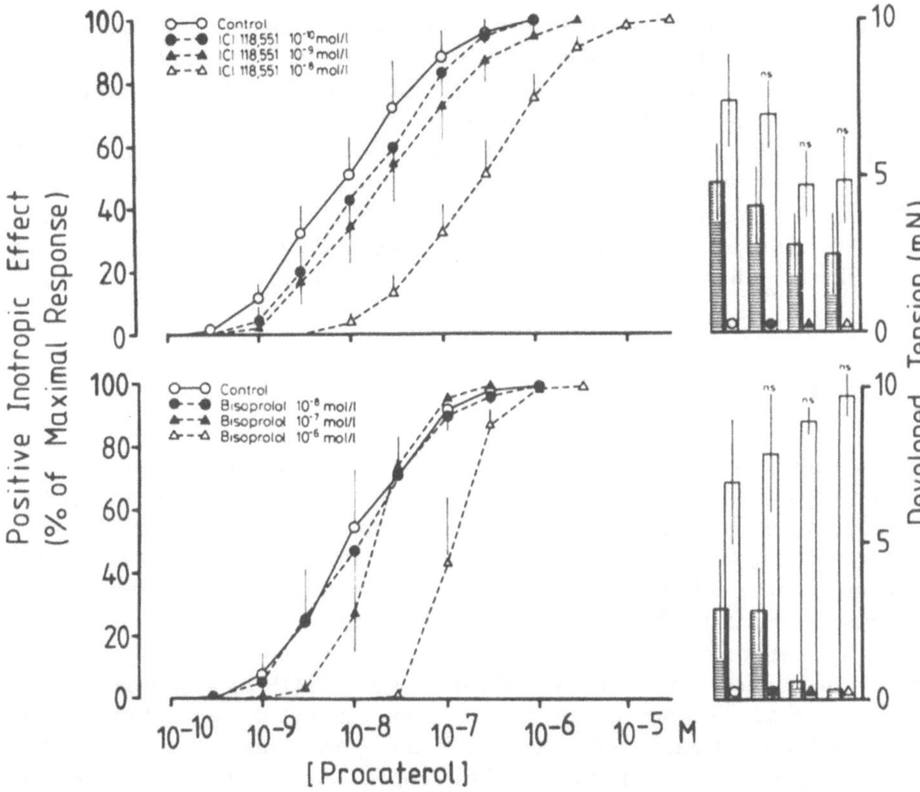

Fig. 7. Influence of ICI 118,551 and bisoprolol respectively on the positive inotropic effect of procaterol on isolated muscle strips of human right atrial appendages. *Left ordinates*, positive inotropic effect as percentage of maximal response; *right ordinates*, basal (▤) and maximal developed tension (□) in the absence and presence of ICI 118,551 and bisoprolol respectively in mN. *Abscissa*, molar concentrations of procaterol. Given are the means ± SEM of six and three experiments respectively. From Zerkowski et al. (1986)

Table 3. Regional distribution of β_1- and β_2-adrenoceptors in the human heart (idiopathic congestive cardiomyopathy)

	β_1/β_2 ratio (%)
Right atrium	62.7 ± 1.9 / 37.3 ± 1.9
Left atrium	66.8 ± 1.4 / 33.2 ± 1.4
Right ventricle	74.4 ± 1.2 / 25.6 ± 1.2
Left ventricle	74.1 ± 1.6 / 25.9 ± 1.6

Given are means ± SEM of three experiments
From Brodde et al. (1986)

tive β_1-antagonist bisoprolol and the highly selective β_2-antagonist ICI 118,551 with the non-subtype-selective radioligand ICYP in human right and left atrium, as well as in right and left ventricular wall obtained from heart transplant recipients who suffered from end-stage heart failure [New York Heart Association (NYHA) class 4]. As shown in Table 3, in all four myocardial tissues investigated, β_1- and β_2-adrenoceptors were identified. The relative amount of β_2-adrenoceptors, however, differed between atria and ventricles: while in both atria, approximately 35% of the β-adrenoceptors were of the β_2-subtype, the amount of β_2-adrenoceptors in the ventricular wall was considerably less (approximately 25%).

Discussion

The first evidence for heterogeneity of β-adrenoceptors in human myocardium was presented by Ablad et al. (1974). They found, on the isolated muscle strip of the right atrial appendage, that the β_1-selective antagonist H 93/26 inhibited the positive inotropic effect of noradrenaline more potently than that of adrenaline, whereas the unselective β-adrenoceptor antagonist propranolol inhibited the responses to both catecholamines to about the same extent. From these results, the authors concluded that human right atria might contain β_1- and β_2-adrenoceptors. This conclusion was supported by experiments performed by Bonelli (1978), who observed that in man, the β-adrenoceptor antagonist mepindolol inhibited the positive chronotropic effect of isoprenaline more potently than its positive inotropic effect. In the present study, we have *directly* identified β_1- and β_2-adrenoceptors in human right atrium by binding studies with the highly specific β-adrenoceptor antagonist radioligand ICYP (Brodde et al. 1981; Engel et al. 1981; Brodde 1982). ICYP binding to membranes from human right atrium was saturable, of high affinity, rapid, reversible and stereospecific. Adrenergic agonists inhibited binding with an order of potency of isoprenaline > adrenaline = noradrenaline, indicating that, in human right atrium, β_1-adrenoceptors predominate. However, inhibition of ICYP binding by β_1- and β_2-selective drugs resulted in shallow displacement curves with pseudo-Hill coefficients which were significantly less than 1.0. Such shallow displacement curves for subtype-selective drugs indicate the existence of a heterogeneous population of β-adrenoceptors (Hoffman and Lefkowitz 1980). Non-linear regression analysis of these displacement curves revealed that human right atria contain approximately 80% β_1- and 20% β_2-adrenoceptors (Table 1). A similar β_1/β_2 ratio has been recently described by Stiles et al. (1983) for human right atrium and by Heitz et al. (1983) for human left atrium.

Both β_1- and β_2-adrenoceptors in human right atrium are functionally coupled to the adenylate cyclase system. Catecholamines stimulated adenylate cyclase activity with a rank order of potency of isoprenaline > adrenaline = noradrenaline, which is identical to that observed for inhibition of ICYP binding. Furthermore, the β_1-selective antagonist betaxolol inhibited isoprenaline-stimulated adenylate cyclase activity much more potently than that activated by the β_2-agonist procaterol. β_2-Adrenoceptors are also involved in β-agonist-induced activation of adenylate cyclase in human right atrium. As shown in Fig. 4, the selective β_2-agonists fenoterol and procaterol stimulated adenylate cyclase activity in a concentration-dependent manner. Their intrinsic activities, however, were only 43%–64% of that of isoprenaline. These effects are mediated by β_2-adrenoceptor stimulation, since the β_2-selective antagonist ICI 118,551 was much more potent in inhibiting procaterol- than isoprenaline-stimulated adenylate cyclase. In addition, the K_{act} values for fenoterol and procaterol for activation of adenylate cyclase were in the same concentration range as their K_I values for inhibition of ICYP binding to β_2-adrenoceptors in human right atrium (Table 2). These results are therefore compatible with the view that procaterol and fenoterol activate human atrial adenylate cyclase via β_2-adrenoceptor stimulation. Thus, there can be no doubt that functional β_1- and β_2-adrenoceptors coexist in human right atrium.

Both β-adrenoceptor subtypes are involved in the positive inotropic action of β-agonists. On the isolated electrically driven human right atrium, the concentration-response curve for the positive inotropic effect of isoprenaline was dose-dependently shifted to the right by the highly selective β_1-adrenoceptor antagonist bisoprolol (10^{-9}–10^{-7} mol/liter); the threshold concentration for bisoprolol was between 10^{-9} and 10^{-8} mol/liter. The dissociation constant for bisoprolol determined either physiologically (Kaumann et al. 1984) or by radioligand binding studies (Wang et al. 1985) is between 3 and 20×10^{-9} mol/liter for β_1-adrenoceptors, while it is approximately 100 times higher (0.2–2.6×10^{-6} mol/liter) for β_2-adrenoceptors. Thus, bisoprolol mainly antagonized the β_1-component of the positive inotropic effect of isoprenaline. However, in the same concentration range, the highly selective β_2-adrenoceptor antagonist ICI 118,551 (10^{-9}–10^{-7} mol/liter) also antagonized the positive inotropic effect of isoprenaline. The dissociation constant for ICI 118,551 at β_2-adrenoceptors determined either physiologically (O'Donnell and Wanstall 1980, 1981; Bilski et al. 1983; Kaumann et al. 1984) or by radioligand binding studies (Dickinson and Nahorski 1981; Brodde et al. 1983) is in the range of 0.3–7×10^{-9} mol/liter, while it is approximately 100 times higher (1–3×10^{-7} mol/liter) at β_1-adrenoceptors. Since the threshold concentration of ICI 118,551 for antagonism of the positive inotropic effect of isoprenaline was between 10^{-9} and 10^{-8} mol/liter, it seems that ICI 118,551 mainly inhibits the β_2-component of isoprenaline. From these results, it can be concluded that, on the isolated electrically driven human right atrium, both β_1- and β_2-adrenoceptors contribute to the positive inotropic action of isoprenaline. This assumption is supported by the fact that for the antagonism of both selective antagonists against isoprenaline the slopes of the Schild plots were significantly less than 1.0, indicating interaction with a heterogeneous population of β-adrenoceptors.

In addition to the unselective β-agonist isoprenaline, the selective β_2-adrenoceptor agonist procaterol produced concentration-dependent increases in force of contraction. Its pD_2 value was 8.03, which corresponds well to the dissociation constant for procaterol at β_2-adrenoceptors determined either physiologically (Yabuuchi 1977; Hedberg and Mattson 1981) or by radioligand binding studies (Hedberg et al. 1980; Brodde et al. 1983). ICI 118,551 shifted the dose-response curve of procaterol to the right in a concentration-dependent manner. In this case, the slope of the Schild plot was not significantly different from 1.0, thus indicating interaction with a homogeneous population of β-adrenoceptors. The pA_2 value for ICI 118,551 was 9.49, which fits very well with the values determined for ICI 118,551 at β_2-adrenoceptors in various organ systems (see above). Accordingly, procaterol mediates its positive inotropic effect on the human right atrium, very likely through stimulation of β_2-adrenoceptors. This is further supported by the fact that bisoprolol was 50–100 times less potent in antagonizing effects of procaterol than in antagonizing those of isoprenaline (Figs. 6 and 7). In addition, the pA_2 value determined for bisoprolol (6.99) was in the same range as that which was determined for β_2-adrenoceptors in various systems. These results clearly demonstrate that β_1- and β_2-adrenoceptors coexist in human right atrial appendage; both are functionally coupled to adenylate cyclase activity and are involved in the positive inotropic responses to β-agonists.

However, β_1- and β_2-adrenoceptors coexist not only in atria, but also in the ventricles. As shown in Table 3, in human right and left atrium and in right and left ventricular wall obtained from heart transplant recipients who suffered from end-stage heart failure, β_1- and β_2-adrenoceptors could be identified. The relative amount of β_2-adrenoceptors, however, differed between atria and ventricles: while in both atria approximately 35% of the β-adrenoceptors were of the β_2-subtype, the amount of β_2-adrenoceptors in the ventricular wall was considerably less (25%). The regional distribution of β_1- and β_2-adrenoceptors in the human myocardium is obviously different from that in the heart of various animal species, where β_2-adrenoceptors could be identified only in the atria but not in the ventricular wall (Hedberg et al. 1980; Minneman et al. 1981; Brodde et al. 1982; Stiles et al. 1984).

The physiological role of β_2-adrenoceptors in the human heart is not known at present. In right atria, they might play a role in regulating heart rate, since it has been shown that, in man, isoprenaline-induced tachycardia could be antagonized to a greater extent by propranolol than by the β_1-selective antagonist atenolol (Brown et al. 1983). Furthermore, Arnold et al. (1985) recently demonstrated that, in man, ICI 118,551 antagonized the isoprenaline-induced tachycardia much more potently than the β_1-selective antagonist atenolol, while propranolol was equipotent to ICI 118,551. The existence of functional β_2-adrenoceptors in left-ventricular myocardium might explain the beneficial effects of the β_2-selective agonist fenoterol in severe heart failure (Irmer et al. 1981), since it has been recently demonstrated that, in fact, fenoterol can increase contractile force in left papillary muscles of the human heart via β_2-adrenoceptor stimulation (Mügge et al. 1985).

Conclusion

In human right atrium, functional β_1- and β_2-adrenoceptors coexist; both β-adrenoceptor subtypes are coupled to the adenylate cyclase system and contribute to the positive inotropic action of catecholamines. In contrast to the heart of various animal species, in the human heart, β_1- and β_2-adrenoceptors coexist in both atria and ventricles; however, the relative amount of β_2-adrenoceptors in the atria (20%–35%) is higher than in the ventricles (15%–25%). The physiological role of β_2-adrenoceptors present in human heart remains to be evaluated.

References

Ablad B, Carlsson B, Carlsson E, Dahlöf C, Ek L, Hultberg F (1974) Cardiac effects of β-adrenergic receptor antagonists. Adv Cardiol 12: 290-302

Arnold JMO, O'Connor PC, Riddell JG, Harron DWG, Shanks RG, McDevitt DG (1985) Effects of the β_2-adrenoceptor antagonist ICI 118,551 on exercise tachycardia and isoprenaline-induced β-adrenoceptor responses in man. Br J Clin Pharmacol 19: 619-630

Arunlakshana O, Schild HO (1959) Some quantitative uses of drug antagonists. Br J Pharmacol 14: 48-58

Bilski AJ, Halliday SE, Fitzgerald JD, Wale JL (1983) The pharmacology of a β_2-selective adrenoceptor antagonist (ICI 118,551). J Cardiovasc Pharmacol 5: 430-437

Bonelli J (1978) Demonstration of two different types of β_1-receptors in man. Int J Clin Pharmacol 16: 313-319

Brodde OE (1982) Homogeneous class of beta-1 adrenergic receptors in rat kidney: identification by (±)-^{125}iodocyanopindolol binding. Biochem Pharmacol 31: 1743-1747

Brodde OE, Engel G, Hoyer D, Bock KD, Weber F (1981) The β-adrenergic receptor in human lymphocytes: subclassification by the use of a new radio-ligand, (±)-^{125}iodocyanopindolol. Life Sci 29: 2189-2198

Brodde OE, Leifert FJ, Krehl HJ (1982) Coexistence of β_1- and β_2-adrenoceptors in the rabbit heart: quantitative analysis of the regional distribution by (–)-^{3}H-dihydroalprenolol binding. J Cardiovasc Pharmacol 4: 34-43

Brodde OE, Karad K, Zerkowski HR, Rohm N, Reidemeister JC (1983) Coexistence of β_1- and β_2-adrenoceptors in human right atrium. Direct identification by (±)-^{125}iodocyanopindolol binding. Circ Res 53: 752-758

Brodde OE, O'Hara N, Zerkowski HR, Rohm N (1984) Human cardiac β-adrenoceptors: both β_1- and β_2-adrenoceptors are functionally coupled to the adenylate cyclase in right atrium. J Cardiovasc Pharmacol 6: 1184-1191

Brodde OE, Schüler S, Kretsch R, Brinkmann M, Borst HG, Hetzer R, Reidemeister JC, Warnecke H, Zerkowski HR (1986) Regional distribution of β-adrenoceptors in the human heart: coexistence of functional β_1- and β_2-adrenoceptors in both atria and ventricles in severe congestive cardiomyopathy. J Cardiovasc Pharmacol in press

Brown JE, McLeod AA, Shand DG (1983) Evidence for cardiac β_2-adrenoceptors in man. Clin Pharmacol Ther 33: 424-428

Carlsson E, Ablad B, Brandstrom A, Carlsson B (1972) Differentiated blockade of the chronotropic effects of various adrenergic stimuli in the cat heart. Life Sci 11: 953-958

Cheng YC, Prusoff WH (1973) Relationship between the inhibition constant (K_i) and the concentration of inhibitor which causes 50 per cent inhibition (I_{50}) of an enzymatic reaction. Biochem Pharmacol 22: 3099-3108

Daly MJ, Levy GP (1979) The subclassification of β-adrenoceptors: evidence in support of the dual β-adrenoceptor hypothesis. In: Kalsner S (ed) Trends in autonomic pharmacology, vol 1. Urban and Schwarzenberg Baltimore, pp 347-382

DeLean A, Hancock AA, Lefkowitz RJ (1982) Validation and statistical analysis of a computer modeling method for quantitative analysis of radioligand binding data for mixtures of pharmacological receptor subtypes. Mol Pharmacol 21: 5-16

Dickinson KEJ, Nahorski SR (1981) Atypical characteristics of frog and chick erythrocyte β-adrenoceptors. Eur J Pharmacol 74: 43-52

Engel G, Hoyer D, Berthold R, Wagner H (1981) (±)-[^{125}]iodocyanopindolol, a new ligand for β-adrenoceptors: identification and quantitation of subclasses of β-adrenoceptors in guinea pig. Naunyn-Schmiedebergs Arch Pharmacol 317: 277-285

Hedberg A, Mattson H (1981) Beta adrenoceptor interaction of full and partial agonists in the cat heart and soleus muscle. J Pharmacol Exp Ther 219: 798-808

Hedberg A, Minneman KP, Molinoff PB (1980) Differential distribution of beta-1 and beta-2 adrenergic receptors in cat and guinea-pig heart. J Pharmacol Exp Ther 212: 503-508

Heitz A, Schwartz J, Velly J (1983) Adrenoceptors of the human myocardium: determination of β_1- and β_2-subtypes by radioligand binding. Br J Pharmacol 80: 711-719

Hoffman BB, Lefkowitz RJ (1980) Radioligand binding studies of adrenergic receptors: new insights into molecular and physiological regulation. Ann Rev Pharmacol Toxicol 20: 581-608

Irmer M, Wollschläger H, Just H (1981) Behandlung der schweren Herzinsuffizienz mit dem Beta-Stimulator Fenoterol. Klin Wochenschr 59: 639-645

Kaumann AJ, Lemoine H, Ehle B (1984) Labeling of heart β_1-adrenoceptors with ^{3}H(–)-bisoprolol and of lung β_2-adrenoceptors with ^{3}H-ICI 118,551. Comparison of affinities estimated from binding and blockade. Naunyn-Schmiedebergs Arch Pharmacol 325 [Suppl R]: 67

Lands AM, Arnold A, McAuliff JP, Luduena FP, Brown TG (1967a) Differentiation of receptor systems activated by sympathomimetic amines. Nature 214: 597-598

Lands AM, Luduena FP, Buzzo HJ (1967b) Differentiation of receptors responsive to isoproterenol. Life Sci 6: 2241-2249

Lefkowitz RJ (1978) Identification and regulation of alpha and beta adrenergic receptors. Fed Proc 37: 123-129

Minneman KP, Hegstrand LR, Molinoff PB (1979) Simultaneous determination of beta-1- and beta-2-adrenergic receptors in tissues containing both receptor subtypes. Mol Pharmacol 16: 34-46

Minneman KP, Pittman RN, Molinoff PB (1981) β-Adrenergic receptor subtypes: properties, distribution and regulation. Ann Rev Neurosci 4: 419-461

Molinoff PB, Wolfe BB, Weiland GA (1981) Quantitative analysis of drug-receptor interactions: II. Determination of the properties of receptor subtypes. Life Sci 29: 427-443

Mügge A, Posselt D, Reimer U, Schmitz W, Scholz H (1985) Effects of the beta$_2$-adrenoceptor agonists fenoterol and salbutamol on force of contraction in isolated human ventricular myocardium. Klin Wochenschr 63: 26-31

O'Donnell SR, Wanstall JC (1980) Evidence that ICI 118,551 is a potent, highly beta$_2$-selective adrenoceptor antagonist and can be used to characterize beta-adrenoceptor populations in tissue. Life Sci 27: 671-677

O'Donnell SR, Wanstall JC (1981) Demonstration of both β_1- and β_2-adrenoceptors mediating relaxation of isolated ring preparations of rat pulmonary artery. Br J Pharmacol 74: 547-552

Scatchard G (1949) The attraction of proteins for small molecules and ions. Ann NY Acad Sci 51: 660-672

Schliep HJ, Harting J (1984) β_1-Selectivity of bisoprolol, a new β-adrenoceptor antagonist, in anesthetized dogs and guinea-pigs. J Cardiovasc Pharmacol 6: 1156-1160

Stiles GL, Taylor S, Lefkowitz RJ (1983) Human cardiac beta-adrenergic receptors: subtype heterogeneity delineated by direct radioligand binding. Life Sci 33: 467-473

Stiles GL, Caron MG, Lefkowitz RJ (1984) β-Adrenergic receptors: biochemical mechanisms of physiological regulation. Physiol Rev 64: 661-743

Van Rossum JM (1963) Cumulative dose-response curves II: technique for the making of dose-response curves in isolated organs and the evaluation of drug parameters. Arch Int Pharmacodyn Ther 143: 299-330

Wang XL, Brinkmann M, Brodde OE (1985) Selective labelling of β_1-adrenoceptors in rabbit lung membranes by (–)-^{3}H-bisoprolol. Eur J Pharmacol 114: 157-165

Yoshizaki S, Tanimura K, Tamada S, Yabuuchi Y, Nakagawa K (1976) Sympathomimetic amines having a carbostyril nucleus. Med Chem 19: 1138-1142

Yabuuchi Y (1977) The β-adrenoceptor stimulant properties of OPC 2009 on guinea-pig isolated tracheal, right atrial and left atrial preparations. Br J Pharmacol 61: 513-521

Zerkowski HR, Ikezono K, Rohm N, Reidemeister JC, Brodde OE (1986) Human myocardial β-adrenoceptors: demonstration of both β_1- and β_2-adrenoceptors mediating contractile responses to β-agonists on the isolated right atrium. Naunyn-Schmiedebergs Arch Pharmacol 332: 142-147.

Effect of Thyroid Hormones on Myocardial Adrenoceptors and Adrenoceptor-Mediated Cardiovascular Responses in the Rat*

G. Groß

Pharmakologisches Institut, Universitätsklinikum Essen, Hufelandstraße 55, 4300 Essen 1, Federal Republic of Germany

Excess and deficiency of thyroid hormones produce distinct changes in cardiovascular responses. Hypothyroidism resembles a "hypoadrenergic state", whereas hyperthyroidism results in tachycardia, increased cardiac output and hypertrophy of the myocardium. These changes have been attributed to alterations in adrenoceptor density and to altered responsiveness to adrenoceptor stimulation of the heart. On the other hand, thyroid hormones seem to exert a complex influence on the release and turnover of noradrenaline (NA) and on plasma catecholamine levels (for review, see Harrison 1964 and Kunos 1981). In this study, thyroid hormone-induced alterations of myocardial α- and β-adrenoceptors were further characterized. The dependence of these adrenoceptor changes on catecholamine availability and some adrenoceptor-mediated cardiovascular responses in dysthyroid states were investigated.

For all experiments, male rats were used. Hypothyroidism was induced by feeding pellets containing 0.18% 6-propyl-2-thiouracil (PTU) for at least 3 weeks, while hyperthyroidism was brought on by daily T_3 injections (500 µg/kg, unless otherwise indicated). The degree of dysthyroid states was checked by plasma T_3 and TSH levels. All values given here represent means ± SEM. Student's and Dunnett's *t* test were used for the comparison of means.

The Effect of Hypo- and Hyperthyroidism on Myocardial Adrenoceptors

The density of β-adrenoceptors in myocardial tissue was determined by [^{3}H]-dihydroalprenolol (^{3}H-DHA) binding. PTU treatment resulted in a significant decrease in the density of ^{3}H-DHA binding sites of the whole heart; artificial hyperthyroidism increased the B_{max} values. The affinity of ^{3}H-DHA to its binding sites remained unchanged by the different treatments (Fig. 1). These observations correspond to earlier reports (Banerjee and Kung 1977; Ciaraldi and Marinetti 1977; Williams et al. 1977; McConnaughy et al. 1979). In contrast to L-T_3 and L-T_4, which are known to be physiologically active, the thyronine derivatives D-T_3 and rT_3 were inactive in this respect, suggesting a specific T_3 receptor-mediated process. The increase in β-adrenoceptor density proved to be dose- and time-dependent and rather rapidly reversible. Daily T_3 doses as low as 10 µg/kg injected i.p. for 8 days induced an in-

* Supported by a grant from the *Deutsche Forschungsgemeinschaft*

New Aspects of the Role of Adrenoceptors in the Cardiovascular System/Ed. by Grobecker et al.

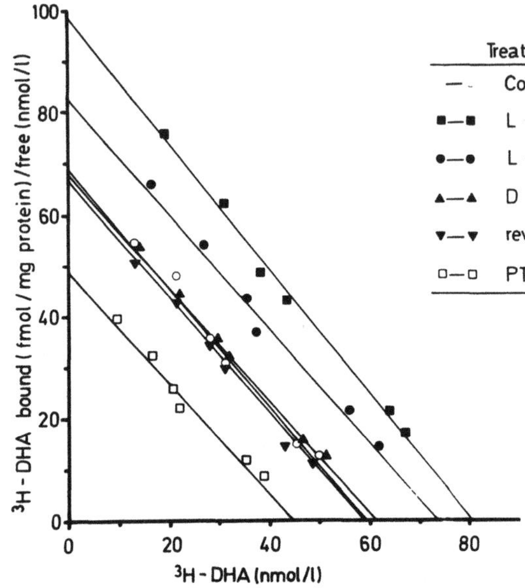

Treatment		N	B_{max} fmol/mg protein	K_D nmol/l
—	Control	9	58.7 ± 2.5	0.87 ± 0.09
■—■	L - T_3	8	78.2 ± 3.3**	0.78 ± 0.03
●—●	L - T_4	7	72.2 ± 6.5*	0.85 ± 0.05
▲—▲	D - T_3	9	60.3 ± 3.3	0.86 ± 0.04
▼—▼	reverse T_3	9	56.5 ± 3.1	0.82 ± 0.02
□—□	PTU	7	42.5 ± 6.1*	0.97 ± 0.08

Fig. 1. Effect of treatment with PTU and iodothyronines on ^{3}H-DHA binding in the rat heart. T_4 and T_3 isomers were injected for 4 days (0.5 µmol/kg per day). Membranes were incubated with 0.25–4 nmol/liter ^{3}H-DHA at 25 °C for 30 min. Unspecific binding was determined in the presence of 1 µmol/liter (−)propanolol. Data are presented as Scatchard plots. * $P<0.05$; ** $P<0.01$ compared with controls

crease in B_{max} values of 34% ($P<0.05$; $n=11$) compared with controls ($n=11$). With a daily dose of 300 µg/kg, a maximum effect (+84%, $P<0.01$; $n=11$) was obtained. A significant T_3-induced increase in ^{3}H-DHA binding sites was already measured after 2 days (+27%; $P<0.05$; $n=6$) and the maximum effect (+66%; $P<0.01$; $n=6$) was reached after 4 days. After discontinuation of T_3 treatment, the number of ^{3}H-DHA binding sites rapidly declined and within 4 days reached the level of euthyroid controls. The loss of ^{3}H-DHA binding sites owing to PTU administration was completely reversible by T_3 injections within 2 days.

In order to decide whether the increase in ^{3}H-DHA binding sites is dependent on protein synthesis, rats were treated with T_3 (500 µg/kg) and cycloheximide (1.5 mg/kg) for 2 days. Cycloheximide alone had no effect on the density of myocardial ^{3}H-DHA binding sites; T_3 alone increased the B_{max} values by 43% ($P<0.01$; $n=8$) as expected, whereas no significant increase in B_{max} values was found in the group concomitantly treated with T_3 and cycloheximide ($P>0.1$; $n=8$). Thus, it appears likely that T_3 increased the density of ^{3}H-DHA binding sites by de novo synthesis of β-adrenoceptors.

The density of α_1-adrenoceptors in myocardial tissue was determined by ^{3}H-prazosin binding. In contrast to β-adrenoceptors, the density of α_1-adrenoceptors in the whole heart decreased as a result of T_3 treatment, as has already been reported by other investigators (Ciaraldi and Marinetti 1977; McConnaughy et al. 1979). However, data as to whether α_1-adrenoceptors increase or decrease in hypothyroidism conflict (for review, see Bilezikian and Loeb 1983). In our experiments, PTU

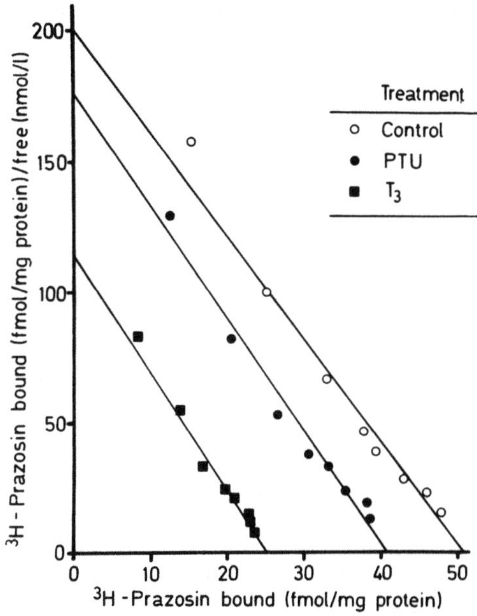

	Treatment	N	B_{max} fmol/mg protein	K_D nmol/l
○	Control	23	52.0 ± 2.4	0.29 ± 0.03
●	PTU	12	41.9 ± 3.2 *	0.28 ± 0.03
■	T_3	12	26.0 ± 2.8 **	0.31 ± 0.07

Fig. 2. Effect of PTU and T_3 treatment on [^{3}H-]prazosin binding in the rat heart. Membranes were incubated with 0.1-4 nmol/liter [^{3}H-]prazosin at 25 °C for 30 min. Unspecific binding was determined in the presence of 1 μmol/liter prazosin. Data are presented as Scatchard plots. * $P<0.05$; ** $P<0.01$ compared with controls

treatment reduced the number of ^{3}H-prazosin binding sites, although not to the same extent as T_3 treatment (Fig. 2). Again, K_D values remained unchanged by both types of treatment.

Since plasma catecholamines and myocardial NA turnover are affected by hypo- and hyperthyroidism respectively (see below), it could not be ruled out that the adrenoceptor changes might be secondary to an altered availability of the endogenous agonists at the receptor sites. However, neither chemical sympathectomy with 6-OH-dopamine (total dose, 500 mg/kg injected over a period of 9 or 23 days, which reduced NA levels in the myocardium by more than 90%) nor adrenalectomy (when an increase in plasma adrenaline level had to be expected) prevented the changes in α_1- and β-adrenoceptor density (Table 1). Hence, these changes cannot be considered as a homologous receptor regulation.

In pithed rats, PTU treatment resulted in a distinct fall in basal heart rate, whereas T_3 treatment (500 μg/kg for 8 days) produced marked tachycardia (Table 2), which could not be reduced to the level of euthyroid controls even by high doses of the β-adrenoceptor antagonists (±)sotalol (10^{-5}mol/kg) and (−)bupranolol (10^{-5}mol/kg). Obviously, the changes in the basal heart rate in dysthyroid states developed independently of the β-adrenoceptor alterations. Isoprenaline (10^{-12}-10^{-8}mol/kg) increased the heart rate of pithed rats by stimulation of β-adrenoceptors. After PTU treatment, the isoprenaline dose-response curve was shifted to the right by more than 0.5 log units, and the maximum response was reduced. This finding is compatible with the reduction in β-adrenoceptor density. On

Table 1. Effect of chemical sympathectomy (6-OH-dopamine) and adrenalectomy on PTU- and T_3-induced changes in myocardial α_1- and β-adrenoceptor binding

Ligand	Treatment	B_{max} (% of the respective control)		
		–	6-OH-dopamine	6-OH-dopamine + adrenalectomy
[^{3}H]-prazosin	Control	100±4	100±8	100±8
	PTU	73±5**		73±7*
	T_3	61±7**	67±4**	
^{3}H-DHA	Control	100±6	100±7	100±4
	PTU	59±6*		77±6*
	T_3	181±8**	157±9**	

* $P<0.05$; ** $P<0.01$, compared with the respective control. $n=7$–16.
6-OH-Dopamine was administered in a total dose of 500 mg/kg before T_3 treatment (5 days) or before and during PTU administration (3 weeks).

In adrenalectomized animals, one adrenal gland was removed, the other one was demedullated. The effect of the different treatments was checked by determination of tissue and plasma catecholamines. Cardiac membranes were incubated with six concentrations of [^{3}H-]prazosin (0.1–3 nmol/liter) and of ^{3}H-DHA (0.1–6 nmol/liter). Unspecific binding was measured in the presence of 1 μmol/liter prazosin and 1 μmol/liter (–)propranolol respectively. The maximal number of binding sites was calculated from Scatchard plots by linear regression analysis

Table 2. Effect of PTU and T_3 treatment on the basal heart rate in pithed and in freely moving rats

Treatment	Heart rate (min^{-1})	
	Pithed rats	Freely moving rats
Control	315±12	323±9
PTU	155± 5*	340±10
T_3 (1 day)	350± 7	400±15*
(2 days)	373±11*	449±18*
(4 days)	408±13*	481±16*
(8 days)	478±13*	

* $P<0.01$ compared with controls; $n=10$–16

the other hand, T_3 treatment had no effect on the ED_{50} value of isoprenaline, but decreased the maximum response (Fig. 3). This may be due to the already considerably enhanced basal heart rate.

T_3 treatment (500 μg/kg for 7 days) produced a significant increase in dry weight of the heart (by 28%; $P<0.01$; $n=10$). This hypertrophy could not be attributed to enhanced β-adrenoceptor stimulation since it was not prevented by 6-OH-dopamine treatment or propranolol (7.5 mg/kg per day administered by osmotic minipumps for 7 days).

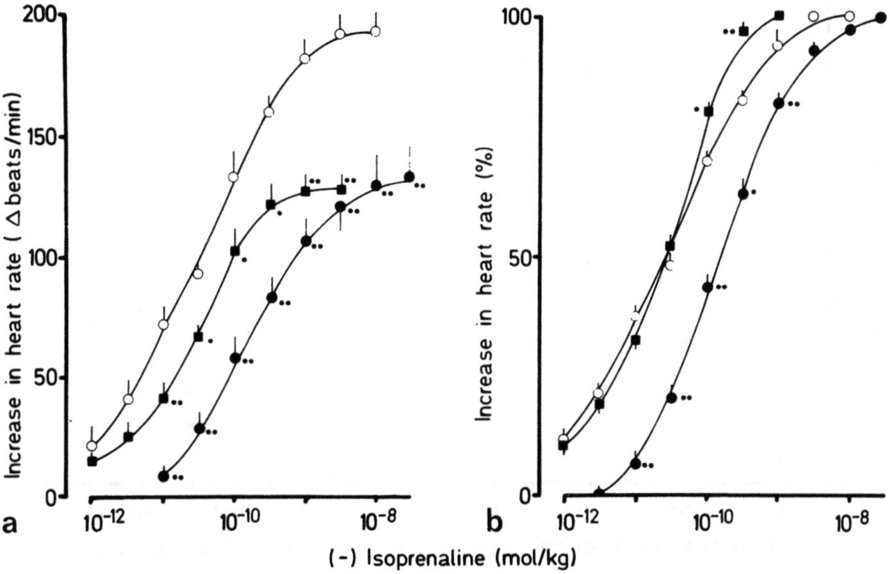

Fig. 3a, b. Effect of PTU and T_3 treatment on the isoprenaline-induced increase in heart rate in pithed rats. Atropine 1.5 mg/kg was administered before the injection of isoprenaline. The heart rate before injection of isoprenaline amounted to $307 \pm 18\ min^{-1}$ in controls ($n = 8$), $178 \pm 10\ min^{-1}$ in the PTU group ($p < 0.01$, $n = 8$), and $474 \pm 21\ min^{-1}$ in the T_3 group ($p < 0.01$, $n = 8$). * $P < 0.05$; ** $P < 0.01$ compared with controls. ○—○, control; ■—■, T_3; ●—●, PTU

The Effect of Hypo- and Hyperthyroidism on Arterial Blood Pressure

In freely moving rats, the mean blood pressure was significantly lowered after PTU administration, but was unaffected by T_3 treatment (controls, 109 ± 5 mm Hg, $n = 10$; PTU group, 94 ± 3 mm Hg, $P < 0.05$, $n = 12$; T_3 group, 101 ± 4, N.S., $n = 12$). The decrease in blood pressure in PTU-treated rats may be partly due to impaired responsiveness of resistance vessels to α-adrenoceptor stimulation. The rise in diastolic blood pressure produced by phenylephrine and 2-amino-6-allyl-5,6,7,8-tetrahydro-4H-thiazolo-[4,5-*d*]-azepine (B-HT 920), predominant α_1- and α_2-adrenoceptor agonists respectively was clearly attenuated in hypothyroid pithed rats (Fig. 4). It is unclear, however, whether this effect is the result of changes in vascular α-adrenoceptors or whether it was caused by alterations in the contractile mechanism. Studies with radioiodinated α-adrenoceptor ligands in vascular tissue would be beneficial for settling this question.

In pithed rats, the PTU-induced decrease in mean blood pressure was even more pronounced than in intact animals (controls, 56 ± 1 mm Hg, $n = 16$; PTU group, 39 ± 1 mm Hg, $P < 0.01$, $n = 14$; T_3 group, 60 ± 2 mm Hg, N.S., $n = 12$). Since there is no sympathetic impulse flow in pithed rats, it appears likely that a reduced cardiac output contributes to the decrease in blood pressure.

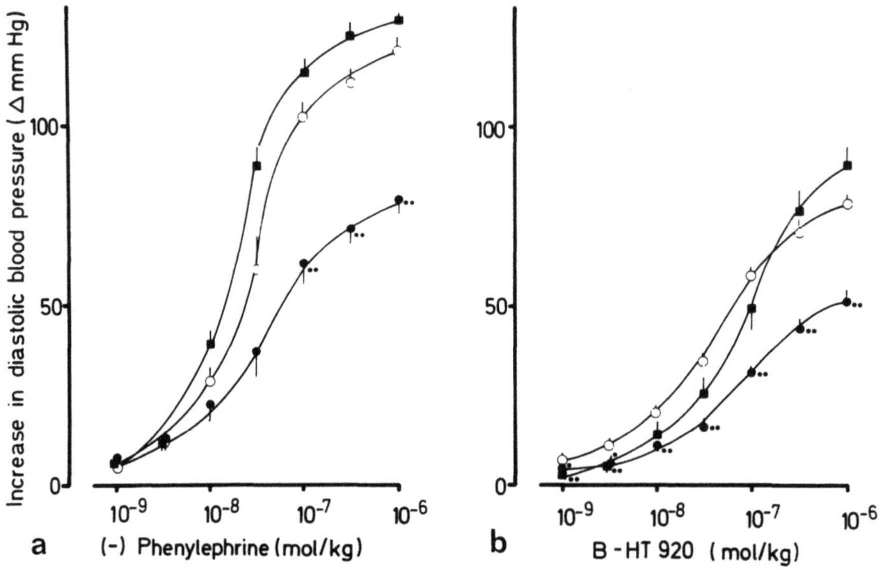

Fig. 4 a, b. Effect of PTU and T_3 treatment on the (−)phenylephrine (**a**)- and B-HT 920 (**b**)-induced increase in diastolic blood pressure in pithed rats. The animals were prepared as described by Schümann et al. (1979). Atropine 1.5 mg/kg and bupranolol 0.3 μmol/kg were administered before the injection of the α-adrenoceptor agonists. The diastolic blood pressure before the injection of phenylephrine and B-HT 920 amounted to 47 ± 1 mm Hg in controls ($n = 12$), 38 ± 3 mm Hg in PTU-treated rats ($P < 0.01$; $n = 10$) and 45 ± 2 mm Hg in T_3-treated rats (N.S.; $n = 10$). * $P < 0.05$; ** $P < 0.01$ compared with controls. ○, control; ■, T_3; ●, PTU

The Effect of Hypo- and Hyperthyroidism on Myocardial and Plasma Catecholamines

T_3 treatment considerably decreased the content and the turnover of noradrenaline in the rat heart. This observation corresponds to the diminished rate of [^{14}C]tyrosine incorporation into catecholamines in the heart and brain of T_4-treated rats communicated by Prange et al. (1970). Landsberg and Axelrod (1968) reported a rise in NA turnover in the hearts of hypophysectomized rats, which they ascribed to TSH as well as ACTH deficiency. In contrast to their observations, we found no significant effect of PTU-induced hypothyroidism on myocardial NA content and turnover (Table 3). In freely moving rats pretreated with PTU, plasma NA and adrenaline levels were increased nine- and five-fold respectively, compared with euthyroid controls. T_3 treatment had no influence on plasma catecholamine levels (Table 4). The marked increase in plasma catecholamines in hypothyroid animals seems to reflect a central nervous mechanism which compensates for the fall in heart rate and blood pressure. Tachycardia in hyperthyroid rats, however, cannot be counteracted by the decrease in myocardial noradrenaline turnover measured in intact animals.

Table 3. Effect of PTU and T_3 treatment on noradrenaline concentration and turnover in the rat heart

Treatment	NA concentration (μg/g)	Rate constant (k) (h^{-1})	$t_{½}$ (h)
Control	0.82 ± 0.04	0.041 ± 0.008	17
PTU	0.90 ± 0.08	0.053 ± 0.011	13
T_3	0.59 ± 0.05*	0.011 ± 0.007*	64

* $P < 0.05$ compared with controls.
NA concentrations were determined radioenzymatically as described by Nagel and Schümann (1980) The parameters of NA turnover were estimated from the loss of endogenous NA after injection of α-methyl-p-tyrosine (300 mg/kg every 3 h) according to Brodie et al. (1966) and Costa (1970). Myocardial NA levels were assayed after 0, 4, 8 and 12 h (n, at least 8 per group at each time check)

Table 4. Effect of PTU and T_3 treatment on plasma catecholamines in freely moving rats

Treatment	NA (pg/ml)	Adrenaline (pg/ml)
Control	161 ± 17	397 ± 81
PTU	1507 ± 178**	1865 ± 716*
T_3 (4 days)	106 ± 38	311 ± 8

* $P < 0.05$, ** $P < 0.01$ compared with controls. $n = 4$–11.
Free plasma catecholamines were determined radioenzymatically (Nagel and Schümann 1980). Blood samples were collected from a catheter implanted into one common carotid artery

Summary

Artificial hypo- and hyperthyroidism in rats induced by feeding PTU and injecting T_3 respectively produce a variety of different effects which contribute to the overall cardiovascular changes. The β-adrenoceptor density in the heart determined by ^{3}H-DHA binding was decreased by PTU and increased by L-T_3 and L-T_4 treatment, whereas D-T_3 and rT_3 were inactive in this respect. The increase in β-adrenoceptors was inhibited by cycloheximide administration, suggesting its dependence on thyroid hormone receptor activation and subsequent protein synthesis. The density of α_1-adrenoceptors in the heart determined by ^{3}H-prazosin binding was reduced in PTU- and even more markedly in T_3-treated animals. The myocardial NA turnover was distinctly decreased by T_3, but remained unaffected by PTU administration. On the other hand, plasma catecholamines were found to be clearly increased by PTU and unaltered by T_3. The changes in myocardial adrenoceptor density proved to come about independently of an altered catecholamine concentration, since they still occurred after chemical sympathectomy and adrenalectomy. The increase in plasma catecholamines measured in freely moving hypothyroid rats compensated for the bradycardia and the fall in blood pressure recorded in hypothyroid pithed rats. The maximal increase in diastolic blood pressure owing to α-adrenoceptor stimulation and the β-adrenoceptor-mediated increase in heart rate were clearly impaired by PTU treatment. The tachycardia and the hypertrophy of the heart in hyperthyroidism did not correlate to the increase in β-adrenoceptor density and the altered availability of catecholamines. It can therefore be concluded that the cardiovascular changes in dysthyroid states can only be explained by a complex interaction of several factors partly independent of the sympathetic nervous system.

Acknowledgements. The skillful technical assistance of Miss U. Jansen, Mrs. A. Sprungmann and Mr. E. Hagelskamp is gratefully acknowledged.

References

Banerjee SP, Kung LS (1977) β-Adrenergic receptors in rat heart: effects of thyroidectomy. Eur J Pharmacol 43: 207-208

Bilezikian JP, Loeb JN (1983) The influence of hyperthyroidism and hypothyroidism on α- and β-adrenergic receptor systems and adrenergic responsiveness. Endocr Rev 4: 378-388

Brodie BB, Costa E, Dlabac A, Neff N, Smookler H (1966) Application of steady state kinetics to the estimation of synthesis rate and turnover time of tissue catecholamines. J Pharmacol Exp Ther 154: 493-498

Ciaraldi T, Marinetti GV (1977) Thyroxine and propylthiouracil effects in vivo on alpha and beta adrenergic receptors in rat heart. Biochem Biophys Res Comm 74: 984-991

Costa E (1970) Simple neuronal models to estimate turnover rate of noradrenergic transmitters in vivo. Biochem Psychopharmacol 2: 169-204

Harrison TS (1964) Adrenal medullary and thyroid relationships. Physiol Rev 44: 161-185

Kunos G (1981) Modulation of adrenergic reactivity and adrenoceptors by thyroid hormones. In: Kunos G (ed) Adrenoceptors and catecholamine action, vol 1. Wiley, New York, pp 298-333

Landsberg L, Axelrod J (1968) Influence of pituitary thyroid and adrenal hormones on norepinephrine turnover and metabolism in the rat heart. Circ Res 22: 559-571

McConnaughy MM, Jones LR, Watanabe AM, Besch HR, Williams LT, Lefkowitz RJ (1979) Thyroxine and propylthiouracil effects on alpha- and beta-adrenergic receptor number, ATPase activities, and sialic acid content of rat cardiac membrane vesicles. J Cardiovasc Pharmacol 1: 609-623

Nagel M, Schümann HJ (1980) A sensitive method for determination of conjugated catecholamines in blood plasma. J Clin Chem Clin Biochem 18: 431-432

Prange AJ Jr, Meek JL, Lipton MA (1970) Catecholamines: diminished rate of synthesis in rat brain and heart after thyroxine pretreatment. Life Sci 9: 901-907

Schümann HJ, Borowski E, Gross G (1979) Changes of adrenoceptor-mediated responses in the pithed rat during propylthiouracil induced hypothyroidism. Eur J Pharmacol 56: 145-152

Williams LT, Lefkowitz RJ, Watanabe AM, Hathaway DR, Besch HR Jr (1977) Thyroid hormone regulation of β-adrenergic receptor number. J Biol Chem 252: 2787-2789

Postsynaptic α-Adrenoceptors in Blood Vessels: Discrepancies Between Results Obtained In Vivo and In Vitro

S. Guimarães

Department of Pharmacology, Medical Faculty, 4200 Porto, Portugal

Introduction

Although the activation of both subtypes of α-adrenoceptors leads to vasoconstriction, they can easily be differentiated according to biochemical, physiological and pharmacological data (Table 1).

Most of the information concerning postsynaptic α-adrenoceptors comes from experiments carried out in vivo; it sometimes does not agree with the information obtained in vitro. There are clear and inevitable differences between in vivo and in vitro conditions which may be responsible for these disagreements. Many local,

Table 1. Some distinctive characteristics of postsynaptic α_1- and α_2-adrenoceptors

α_1-Adrenoceptor-mediated effect	α_2-Adrenoceptor-mediated effect
Preferentially evoked by phenylephrine[a] and methoxamine[a]	Preferentially evoked by clonidine[a] and oxymetazoline[a]
Preferentially antagonized by prazosin[b] and phenoxybenzamine[c]	Preferentially antagonized by yohimbine[d] and rauwolscine[e]
Quicker response[f]	Slower response[f]
Independent of extracellular calcium (in vivo)[g]	Dependent on extracellular calcium (in vivo)[g]
Does not require corticosteroid[h]	Requires corticosteroid[h]
Unaffected by strychnine-induced hyperpolarization[i]	Antagonized by strychnine-induced hyperpolarization[i]
Enhanced by warming[j]	Antagonized by warming[j]
Increased turnover of phosphatidylinositol[k]	Inhibition of adenylate cyclase[k]

[a] Starke (1972); Starke et al. (1974); Starke et al. (1975a).
[b] Cambridge et al. (1977).
[c] Dubocovich and Langer (1974).
[d] Starke et al. (1975b).
[e] Tanaka et al. (1978).
[f] McGrath (1983).
[g] Van Meel et al. (1981).
[h] Van Meel et al. (1982).
[i] G. Haeusler (personal communication).
[j] Cooke et al. (1984).
[k] Fain and Garcia-Sainz (1980).

New Aspects of the Role of Adrenoceptors in the Cardiovascular System/Ed. by Grobecker et al.

nervous and humoral factors ocurring in vivo determine the resistance of the vascular beds and can change the blood supply, and the ionic and metabolic phenomena. These can explain the differences in results obtained in these two different "ecological" conditions.

It is well known that respiratory acidosis can cause a switch in the pressor effect of adrenaline from α_1- to α_2-adrenoceptors (McGrath 1983); moreover, the renin-angiotensin-aldosterone system exclusively influences vascular tone owing to α_2-adrenoceptors (De Jonge et al. 1981). On the other hand, it was shown in vitro that angiotensin may convert atypical α_2-adrenoceptors to those which are typical (Schümann and Lues 1983).

With the aim of further characterizing both subtypes of postsynaptic α-adrenoceptors, I should like to mention and discuss the discrepancies between results obtained in vivo and in vitro relative to the following points: (a) the apparent relevance of postsynaptic α-adrenoceptor subtypes; (b) the distribution of postsynaptic α-adrenoceptor subtypes in relation to the sympathetic nerve endings; (c) the intrinsic activity at both subtypes of α-agonists; (d) calcium channel blockers and the activation of postsynaptic α-adrenoceptor subtypes.

The Apparent Relevance of Postsynaptic α-Adrenoceptor Subtypes

The existence of two different subgroups of postsynaptic α-adrenoceptors in blood vessels was postulated on the basis of results obtained in experiments performed in vivo (Drew and Whiting 1979; Docherty et al. 1979; Timmermans et al. 1979). The first results supporting this hypothesis came from experiments carried out on the whole animal. Confirmatory observations were then made in more restricted vascular areas, such as isolated hind limb preparations (Kobinger and Pichler 1980; Madjar et al. 1980; Gardiner and Peters 1982) and the renal (Horn et al. 1982), femoral (Horn et al. 1982) and mesenteric circulation (Shepperson et al. 1982).

In contrast to the ease with which confirmatory evidence for the existence of two subgroups of α-adrenoceptors was obtained in vivo, it was relatively difficult to demonstrate postsynaptic α_2-adrenoceptors in vitro (De Mey and Vanhoutte 1980; Shoji et al. 1983).

This prompted us to compare the distribution of postsynaptic α-adrenoceptor subgroups in five different vascular beds of the dog in vivo (internal carotid, splenic, mesenteric, renal and femoral) with that of in vitro arteries belonging to the same vascular circuits (Guimarães and Garrett 1982; Polónia et al. 1985; Polónia et al. 1986). The results obtained in vivo show that, in all vascular beds, there are both postsynaptic α_1- and α_2-adrenoceptors, although the relative contribution of the two populations of α-adrenoceptors to the pressor response varied from bed to bed: in the renal and splenic vascular beds, α_1-adrenoceptors predominate (more markedly in the renal vascular bed than in that of the spleen), while in the internal carotid, femoral and mesenteric circulation, α_2-adrenoceptors seem to predominate. However, the results obtained in experiments carried out in vitro with strips of arterial vessels belonging to the same vascular beds of the same animal species (renal, splenic, femoral, jejunal and cranial mesenteric arteries of the dog) showed that only α_1-adrenoceptors are present postsynaptically in any of the five arterial vessels studied (Polónia et al. 1985).

Can this discrepancy between results obtained in vivo and in vitro be ascribed to the existence of α_2-adrenoceptors in veins which might account for the pressor responses caused by the α_2-adrenoceptor agonists in vivo? Shoji et al. (1983) obtained evidence in favour of the existence of postsynaptic α_2-adrenoceptors in several veins of the dog, and Gerold and Haeusler (1983) reported cardiac output increases caused by clonidine and 2-amino-6-allyl-5,6,7,8-tetrahydro-4*H*-thiazolo-[4,5-*d*]azepine (B-HT 920) in the pithed rat. If the increase in cardiac output reflected venous constriction, then one could accept the theory that α_2-adrenoceptor activation in veins may account for the pressor responses elicited by α_2-adrenoceptor agonists in vivo and that it may be the cause of this discrepancy between results in vivo and in vitro.

It is also possible that α_2-adrenoceptors are associated only with the arterioles which regulate the peripheral resistance observed in vivo and which are not available for studies in vitro (Docherty and Starke 1981).

Another possible explanation is that α_2-adrenoceptors lose their reactivity following some alterations occurring in the absence of humoral factors. De Jonge et al. (1981) showed that captopril selectively impairs vasoconstriction subserved in vivo by postsynaptic α_2-adrenoceptors, indicating that the renin-angiotensin-aldosterone system influences α_2-adrenoceptor activation in vivo. Furthermore, it has been shown in vitro that the postsynaptic α_2-adrenoceptors of the rabbit saphenous vein require the blood-borne substance angiotensin for their expression (Schümann and Lues 1983; Lues and Schümann 1984).

The Distribution of Postsynaptic α-Adrenoceptor Subtypes in Relation to the Sympathetic Nerve Terminals

Based on the differences in the effectiveness of several α-adrenoceptor antagonists in inhibiting the pressor responses to sympathetic stimulation and to exogenous noradrenaline in pithed rats, Yamaguchi and Kopin (1980) suggested that the pressor effects of exogenous catecholamines are mediated predominantly by α_2-adrenoceptors. They also proposed that the response to sympathetic stimulation is the result of activation of α_1-adrenoceptors in the region of the vascular neuro-effector junction. Confirmatory results were obtained by Langer and Shepperson (1982) in the autoperfused hind limb of the dog, the isolated perfused cat spleen and the cat in vivo where vasoconstriction caused by nerve stimulation and phenylephrine is inhibited by prazosin and the vasoconstrictor response to exogenous noradrenaline is not. A similar conclusion was reached by Wilffert et al. (1982): postsynaptic α_2-adrenoceptors are mainly found extrajunctionally and are sensitive to exogenous noradrenaline or circulating adrenaline, whereas α_1-adrenoceptors are located mainly at the neuro-effector junction and are sensitive to endogenous noradrenaline.

At the same time, we showed in experiments with the dog saphenous vein in vitro that α_2-adrenoceptors are situated closer to the nerve terminals than are α_1-adreno-

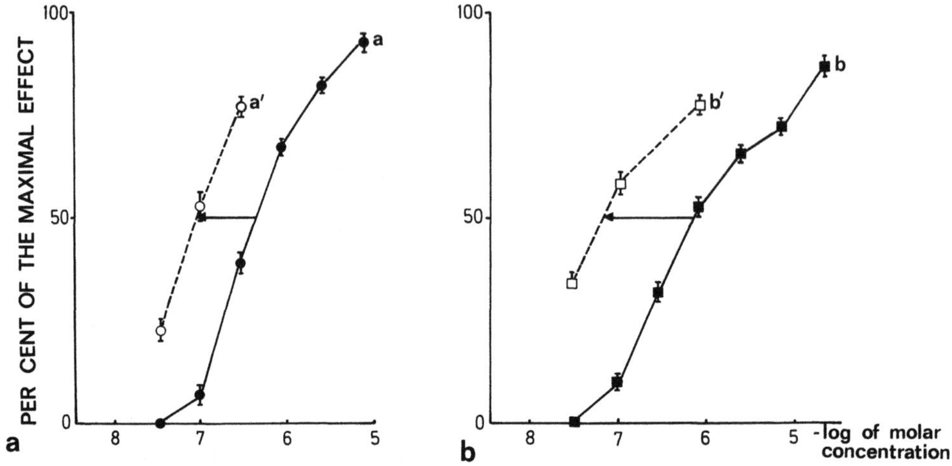

Fig. 1 a, b. Dog saphenous vein. Shown are the concentration-response curves for noradrenaline determined in the presence of 0.5 μmol/liter propranolol and 50 μmol/liter U-0521.
a Curves obtained in the presence of 20 nmol/liter yohimbine; **b** Curves obtained in the presence of 56 nmol/liter prazosin. Between *a* and *a'* and *b* and *b'*, cocaine (12 μmol/liter) was added to the bath

Table 2. Antagonism exerted by prazosin and yohimbine against the responses caused by noradrenaline, electrical stimulation and tyramine

Vasoconstrictor stimulus	pA_2 of antagonism exerted by			
	Prazosin	*n*	Yohimbine	*n*
Noradrenaline	7.57 ± 0.05 (*a*)	15	7.85 ± 0.05 (*d*)	15
Electrical stimulation	6.74 ± 0.07 (*b*)	8	7.95 ± 0.09 (*e*)	8
Tyramine	7.45 ± 0.12 (*c*)	10	8.64 ± 0.09 (*f*)	10

Shown are arithmetic means ± SE. Significant were the differences between: (*a*) and (*b*) ($P < 0.01$); (*b*) and (*e*) ($P < 0.001$); (*c*) and (*f*) ($P < 0.001$)

ceptors (Guimarães et al. 1983). After demonstrating that responses to noradrenaline in the presence of 56 nmol/liter prazosin are exclusively, or at least predominantly, α_2-adrenoceptor-mediated and that responses to noradrenaline in the presence of 20 nmol/l yohimbine are exclusively, or at least predominantly, α_1-adrenoceptor-mediated, we compared, in both situations, the influence of inhibition of neuronal uptake (by cocaine) on the responses of the vein strips to noradrenaline. We observed that cocaine caused an approximately ten-fold increase in sensitivity to noradrenaline in the presence of prazosin, but only an approximately five-fold increase in the presence of yohimbine (Fig. 1). The sensitivity to noradrenaline was the same in either the presence of prazosin or in that of yohimbine. Hence, there is no danger that neuronal uptake was saturated more in one experiment than in the other one. Moreover, yohimbine was more potent than prazosin as an antagonist of the effect caused by noradrenaline released from nerve terminals either by electrical stimulation or by tyramine (Table 2). My conclusion is that - in contrast to the in vivo experiments - α_2-adrenoceptors are closer to the nerve endings than are α_1-adrenoceptors.

A similar conclusion was reached by Cooke et al. (1984) in experiments carried out on the same tissue of the same animal species and by Docherty and Hyland (1984) in experiments carried out on the human saphenous vein. This discrepancy between results obtained in vivo and in vitro can be due at least in part to the different distribution of the sympathetic nerve endings. These nerve endings are evenly distributed throughout the media in the dog saphenous vein and asymmetrically distributed at the adventitio-medial junction in the arteries (Osswald and Guimarães 1983). They are perhaps also asymmetrically distributed in the small arterioles, which are responsible for the blood or perfusion pressure changes in experiments in vivo.

The Intrinsic Activity of both Subtypes of α-Adrenoceptor Agonists

Are α_2-adrenoceptor stimulants partial or full agonists? Perhaps because of the difficulty in obtaining maximal responses, no clear indication on this subject has resulted from investigations carried out in vivo. In contrast, there is no doubt that the maximal responses caused by α_2-adrenoceptor agonists in vitro are smaller than those caused by selective α_1-adrenoceptor agonists or by noradrenaline (a non-selective α_1- and α_2-adrenoceptor agonist). However, this fact does not allow one to conclude that α_2-adrenoceptor stimulants are partial agonists.

To study this problem, we compared - in the dog saphenous vein, a tissue where postsynaptic α_1- and α_2-adrenoceptors coexist - the maximal responses to clonidine and 5-bromo-6-(2-imidazolin-2-ylamino)-quinoxaline (UK-14304) with those to phenylephrine and noradrenaline. We also compared the maximal responses to noradrenaline in the presence of prazosin with those to noradrenaline in the presence of yohimbine. Figure 2 shows the concentration-response curves obtained under the different conditions.

The most interesting feature is that the concentration-response curve for noradrenaline in the presence of prazosin (α_2-adrenoceptor-mediated; Fig. 2B) is biphasic and its first part - that before it becomes steeper - resembles the concentration-response curve for UK-14304: they are parallel and have a similar maximum. It is also worth noting that the point where the curve becomes steeper is shifted to the right (at the same height) when the concentration of prazosin increases, i.e. the increase in concentration of prazosin causes a parallel displacement to the right of the curve, which maintains its biphasic shape. This demonstrates that, when noradrenaline acts only on postsynaptic α_2-adrenoceptors, it causes a maximal effect which is like that which is produced by the selective α_2-adrenoceptor agonist UK-14304 and is smaller than the maximal effect produced by activation of α_1-adrenoceptors, either by phenylephrine or by noradrenaline in the presence of yohimbine. Hence, it may be concluded that UK-14304 and clonidine are full agonists, since they produce the maximally possible effect produced through activation of α_2-adrenoceptors.

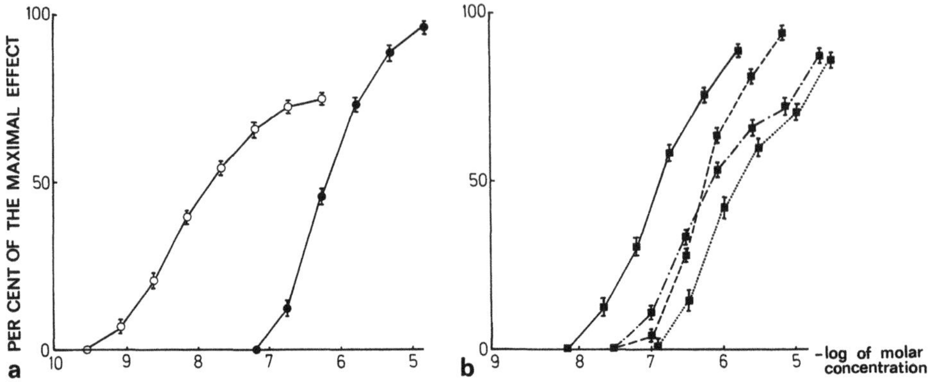

Fig. 2 a, b. Dog saphenous vein. Concentration-response curves for the contractions caused by α-adrenoceptor stimulants. All curves were determined in the presence of 12 µmol/liter cocaine, 0.5 µmol/liter propranolol and 50 µmol/liter U-0521. **a** ○—○ Concentration-response curve for UK-14304 ($n=8$); ●—● concentration response curve for phenylephrine ($n=8$). **b** ■—■ Concentration-response curve for noradrenaline ($n=14$); ■---■ concentration-response curve for noradrenaline in the presence of 20 nmol/liter yohimbine ($n=7$); ■-·-·-■ concentration-response curve for noradrenaline in the presence of 56 nmol/liter prazosin ($n=7$); ■·····■ concentration-response curve for noradrenaline in the presence of 168 nmol/liter prazosin ($n=3$)

Calcium Channel Blockers and the Activation of Postsynaptic α-Adrenoceptor Subtypes

Another differentiating feature of postsynaptic vascular α_1- and α_2-adrenoceptors is the susceptibility of responses of each receptor subtype to antagonism by calcium channel blockers. There is now evidence that the contractile mechanism in vascular smooth muscle involves both influx of extracellular calcium and release of intracellular calcium and that the relative dependence of the contraction on these two calcium sources varies among blood vessels and species studied.

On the basis of data obtained in pithed animals, some investigators have suggested that α_2-adrenoceptor-mediated vasoconstriction depends on the influx of extracellular calcium, while vasoconstriction due to α_1-adrenoceptor activation is not governed by an influx of calcium (Van Meel et al. 1981; Gerold and Haeusler 1983; Van Zwieten et al. 1983).

In contrast to this conclusion based on the invariable susceptibility to inhibition by calcium channel blockers of vasoconstriction triggered by α_2-adrenoceptor activation in in vivo experiments, no clear relationship has been established between calcium channel blockers and vasoconstriction due to α-adrenoceptor activation obtained in vitro.

The relative dependence on release of intracellular calcium or influx of extracellular calcium of α_1- and α_2-adrenoceptor-mediated effects in vitro was first reported by De Mey and Vanhoutte (1980). The authors observed that, in isolated canine splenic arteries and saphenous veins, the α_1-adrenoceptor agonist methoxamine caused contractions which were more sensitive to verapamil than those produced by noradrenaline, a non-selective α-adrenoceptor agonist. Subsequent studies in isolated dog coronary arteries indicated that responses to α_1-adrenoceptor activation were almost completely dependent upon extracellular calcium (Rimele et al. 1983). However, using the isolated dog saphenous vein, Langer and Shepperson (1982) observed that the contraction due to α_2-adrenoceptor activation was markedly reduced by diltiazem, whereas the response to α_1-adrenoceptor activation was only slightly reduced by this drug. Godfraind et al. (1982) arrived at a similar conclusion, since they demonstrated that a selective α_2-adrenoceptor agonist failed to elicit any release of intracellular calcium.

More recently, in the isolated rat aorta and mesenteric artery, which are two vessels possessing exclusively postsynaptic α_1-adrenoceptors, Cauvin and Malik (1984) observed that the α_1-selective antagonist prazosin was about 1000-fold more potent in inhibiting noradrenaline-induced intracellular calcium release and influx of extracellular calcium than was yohimbine. On the other hand, yohimbine inhibition of noradrenaline-evoked intracellular calcium release was not significantly different from its inhibition of noradrenaline-evoked calcium entry. These data show that α_1-adrenoceptor activation promotes both calcium influx and intracellular calcium release in these two isolated rat vessels, as was previously shown in isolated rabbit aorta, another tissue possessing only postsynaptic α_1-adrenoceptors (Cauvin et al. 1982); a discrepancy is evident between results obtained in vivo and in vitro.

However, it has been suggested, on the basis of results obtained in vivo, that the differential antagonism by calcium channel blockers of the responses mediated by vascular α_1- and α_2-adrenoceptors might be related to differences in receptor reserve (spare receptors) between the postsynaptic vascular α-adrenoceptor subtypes (Hamilton et al. 1983). This hypothesis was also adopted by Ruffolo and Yaden (1984), who showed that α_1-adrenoceptors possess a five-fold greater receptor reserve than do α_2-adrenoceptors. Hence, non-competitive antagonists, such as the calcium channel blockers, might inhibit α_2-adrenoceptor-mediated vasoconstriction to a greater extent than α_1-adrenoceptor-mediated responses, even if both processes were equally dependent upon influx of extracellular calcium, since non-competitive antagonists produce greater inhibition in systems lacking a receptor reserve than in those with a receptor reserve (Ariëns and Van Rossum 1957). Subsequently, Ruffolo et al. (1984) reported that, after removal of spare postsynaptic vascular α_1-adrenoceptors by treatment with low doses of phenoxybenzamine (an irreversible α-adrenoceptor antagonist), the pressor response to cirazoline - which the authors consider to act on α_1-adrenoceptors - became highly sensitive to antagonism by diltiazem, resembling α_2-adrenoceptor-mediated vasoconstriction for which no receptor reserve exists.

If responses to cirazoline after treatment with phenoxybenzamine were really α_1-adrenoceptor-mediated (unfortunately, the influence exerted by α_2-adrenoceptor-blocking drugs on this effect of cirazoline after phenoxybenzamine has not been checked), then a good bridge would connect results obtained in vivo and in vitro, overcoming at least in part the discrepancy we referred to.

Final Comment

The discovery of discrepancies is always welcome. When discrepancies arise between results obtained in vivo and in vitro, they sometimes reflect real consequences of the different biological backgrounds and they will persist, even after having been explained. Sometimes discrepancies are due to different technical or methodological approaches and can be resolved. However, discrepancies sometimes appear because authors prefer to give priority to publishing results rather than to accuracy in obtaining them. Thus, the speed with which these questions are clarified often depends on the importance of the subject and on the prestige of the author.

References

Ariëns EJ, Van Rossum JM (1957) pD_x, pA_x and pD'_x values in the analysis of pharmacodynamics. Arch Int Pharmacodyn Ther 110: 275-299

Cambridge D, Davey MJ, Massingham R (1977) Prazosin, a selective antagonist of post-synaptic α-adrenoceptors. Br J Pharmacol 59: 514P-515P

Cauvin C, Malik S (1984) Induction of Ca^{++} influx and intracellular Ca^{++} release in isolated rat aorta and mesenteric resistance vessels by norepinephrine activation of alpha-1 receptors. J Pharmacol Exp Ther 230: 413-418

Cauvin C, Loutzenhiser R, Hwang O, Van Breemen C (1982) α_1-adrenoceptors induce Ca influx and intracellular Ca release in isolated rabbit aorta. Eur J Pharmacol 84: 233-235

Cooke JP, Shepherd JT, Vanhoutte PM (1984) The effect of warming on adrenergic neurotransmission in canine cutaneous vein. Circ Res 54: 547-553

De Jonge A, Wilffert B, Kalkman HO, Van Meel JCA, Thoolen MJMC, Timmermans PBMWM, Van Zwieten PA (1981) Captopril impairs the vascular smooth muscle contraction mediated by postsynaptic α_2-adrenoceptors in the pithed rat. Eur J Pharmacol 74: 385-386

De Mey JG, Vanhoutte PM (1980) Differences in pharmacological properties of postjunctional alpha-adrenergic receptors among arteries and veins. Arch Int Pharmacodyn Ther 244: 328-329

Docherty JR, Hyland L (1984) Neuro-effector transmission through postsynaptic α_2-adrenoceptors in human saphenous vein. Br J Pharmacol 83: 362P

Docherty JR, Starke K (1981) Postsynaptic α-adrenoceptor subtypes mediating nerve-evoked contractions in rabbit blood vessels in vitro. Br J Pharmacol 74: 803P

Docherty JR, MacDonald AM, McGrath JC (1979) Further sub-classification of α-adrenoceptors in the cardiovascular system, vas deferens and anococcygeus of the rat. Br J Pharmacol 67: 421P-422P

Drew GM, Whiting SB (1979) Evidence for two distinct types of postsynaptic α-adrenoceptors in vascular smooth muscle in vivo. Br J Pharmacol 67: 207-215

Dubocovich ML, Langer SZ (1974) Negative feedback regulation of noradrenaline release by nerve stimulation in the perfused cat's spleen: differences in potency of phenoxybenzamine in blocking the pre- and post-synaptic receptors. J Physiol (Lond) 237: 505-519

Fain JN, Garcia-Sainz JA (1980) Role of phosphatidylinositol turnover in $alpha_1$ and of adenylate cyclase inhibition in $alpha_2$ effects of catecholamines. Life Sci 26: 1183-1194

Gardiner JC, Peters CJ (1982) Postsynaptic α_1- and α_2-adrenoceptor involvement in the vascular responses to neuronally released and exogenous noradrenaline in the hindlimb of the dog and cat. Eur J Pharmacol 84: 189-198

Gerold M, Haeusler G (1983) α_2-Adrenoceptors in rat resistance vessels. Naunyn-Schmiedebergs Arch Pharmacol 322: 29-33

Godfraind T, Miller RC, Lima JS (1982) Selective α_1- and α_2-adrenoceptor agonist induced contractions and ^{45}Ca fluxes in the rat isolated aorta. Br J Pharmacol 77: 596-604

Guimarães S, Garrett J (1982) Postsynaptic alpha-adrenoceptor subtypes in five different vascular beds of the dog. Naunyn-Schmiedebergs Arch Pharmacol 321 [Suppl]: R65
Guimarães S, Paiva MQ, Polónia JJ (1983) Alpha$_1$- and alpha$_2$-adrenoceptors of the dog saphenous vein and their relation to the sympathetic nerve terminals. Progr Neuropsychopharmacol Biol Psychiatry (Abstracts) [Suppl]: 155
Hamilton CA, Reid JR, Summer DJ (1983) Acute effects of phenoxybenzamine on α-adrenoceptor response in vivo and in vitro: Relation of in vivo pressor responses to the number of specific adrenoceptor binding sites. J Cardiovasc Pharmacol 5: 868-873
Horn PT, Kohli JD, Listinsky JJ, Goldberg LI (1982) Regional variation in the alpha-adrenergic receptors in the canine resistance vessels. Naunyn-Schmiedebergs Arch Pharmacol 318: 166-172
Kobinger W, Pichler L (1980) Investigations into different types of post-and presynaptic α-adrenoceptors at cardiovascular sites in rats. Eur J Pharmacol 65: 393-402
Langer SZ, Shepperson NB (1982) Recent developments in vascular smooth muscle pharmacology: the post-synaptic α_2-adrenoceptor. Trends in Pharmacol Sci 3: 440-444
Lues I, Schümann HJ (1984) B-HT 920 acts as an α_1-adrenoceptor agonist in the rabbit aorta under certain in vitro conditions. Naunyn-Schmiedebergs Arch Pharmacol 325: 42-46
Madjar H, Docherty JR, Starke K (1980) An examination of pre- and postsynaptic α-adrenoceptors in the autoperfused rabbit hindlimb. J Cardiovasc Pharmacol 2: 619-627
McGrath JC (1983) The variety of vascular α-adrenoceptors. Trends in Pharmacol Sci 4: 14-18
Osswald W, Guimarães S (1983) Adrenergic mechanisms in blood vessels: morphological and pharmacological aspects. Rev Physiol Biochem Pharmacol 96: 53-122
Polónia JJ, Paiva MQ, Guimarães S (1985) Pharmacological characterization of postsynaptic α-adrenoceptor subtypes in five different dog arteries in vitro. J Pharm Pharmacol 37: 205-208
Polónia JJ, Guerreiro M, Guimarães S, Garrett J (1986) Postsynaptic α-adrenoceptor subtypes in the internal carotid, mesenteric, splenic, renal and femoral vascular beds of the dog. Arch Int Pharmacodyn Ther 279: 5-16
Rimele JT, Rooke TW, Aahrus LL, Vanhoutte PM (1983) Alpha$_1$-adrenoceptors in calcium in isolated canine coronary arteries. J Pharmacol Exp Ther 226: 668-672
Ruffolo RR, Yaden EL (1984) Existence of spare α_1-adrenoceptors, but not α_2-adrenoceptors, for respective vasopressor effects of cirazoline and B-HT 933 in the pithed rat. J Cardiovasc Pharmacol 6: 1011-1019
Ruffolo RR, Morgan EL, Messik K (1984) Possible relationship between receptor reserve and the differential antagonism of alpha-1- and alpha-2-adrenoceptor-mediated pressor responses by calcium channel antagonists in the pithed rat. J Pharmacol Exp Ther 230: 587-594
Schümann HJ, Lues I (1983) Postjunctional α-adrenoceptors in the isolated saphenous vein of the rabbit. Characterization and influence of angiotensin. Naunyn-Schmiedebergs Arch Pharmacol 323: 328-334
Shepperson NB, Duval N, Langer SZ (1982) Dopamine decreases mesenteric blood flow in the anaesthetized dog through the stimulation of postsynaptic α_2-adrenoceptors. Eur J Pharmacol 81: 627-635
Shoji T, Tsuru H, Shigei T (1983) A regional difference in the distribution of postsynaptic alpha-adrenoceptor subtypes in canine veins. Naunyn-Schmiedebergs Arch Pharmacol 324: 246-255
Starke K (1972) α-Sympathomimetic inhibition of adrenergic and cholinergic transmission in the rabbit heart. Naunyn-Schmiedebergs Arch Pharmacol 274: 18-45
Starke K, Montel H, Gayk W, Merker R (1974) Comparison of the effects of clonidine on pre- and postsynaptic adrenoceptors in the rabbit pulmonary artery. Naunyn-Schmiedebergs Arch Pharmacol 285: 133-150
Starke K, Endo T, Taube HD (1975 a) Pre- and postsynaptic components in effect of drugs with α-adrenergic affinity. Nature 254: 440-441
Starke K, Montel H, Gayk W, Merker R (1975 b) Preferential blockade of presynaptic α-adrenoceptors by yohimbine. Eur J Pharmacol 34: 385-388
Tanaka T, Weitzell R, Starke K (1978) High selectivity of rauwolscine for presynaptic α-adrenoceptors. Eur J Pharmacol 52: 239-240
Timmermans PBMWM, Kwa HY, Van Zwieten PA (1979) Possible subdivision of postsynaptic α-adrenoceptors mediating pressor response in the pithed rat. Naunyn-Schmiedebergs Arch Pharmacol 310: 189-193
Van Meel JCA, DeJonge A, Kalkman KO, Wilffert B, Timmermans PBMWM, Van Zwieten PA

(1981) Vascular smooth muscle contraction initiated by postsynaptic α_2-adrenoceptor activation is induced by an influx of extracellular calcium. Eur J Pharmacol 69: 205–208

Van Meel JCA, Wilffert B, Kalkman HO, Thoolen MJMC, De Jonge A, Timmermans PBMWM, Van Zwieten PA (1982) α_2-adrenergic pressor responses and corticosteroids in the pithed rat. Br J Pharmacol 75: 137P

Van Zwieten PA, Van Meel JCA, Timmermans PBMWM (1983) Functional interaction between calcium antagonists and the vasoconstriction induced by the stimulation of postsynaptic α_2-adrenoceptors. Cir Res 52 [Suppl 1]: 177–180

Wilffert B, Timmermans PBMWM, Van Zwieten PA (1982) Extrasynaptic location of alpha-2 and noninnervated beta-2 adrenoceptors in the vascular system of the pithed normotensive rat. J Pharmacol Exp Ther 221: 762–768

Yamaguchi I, Kopin IJ (1980) Differential inhibition of alpha-1 and alpha-2 adrenoceptor-mediated pressor responses in pithed rats. J Pharmacol Exp Ther 214: 275–281

Adrenaline Reversal and Postjunctional α-Adrenoceptors

W. Osswald and E. Rodrigues-Pereira

Department of Pharmacology, Faculty of Medicine, 4200 Porto, Portugal

Adrenaline Reversal: Early Observations and Interpretations

In his seminal paper of 1906, Dale, in describing vasomotor reversal caused by an impure ergot preparation, observed that the pressor response to adrenaline was reversed to a depressor response, but that relaxation of the uterus, also brought about by adrenaline, remained unaltered. Dale concluded that "paralysis of the normally preponderant motor elements allows the emergence of a normally masked inhibitor effect".

The vast amount of experience gathered with other, more potent and more specific adrenergic-blocking drugs confirmed and extended Dale's observations. It was therefore only logical, once Ahlquist (1948) had established the division in α- and β-adrenoceptors, to adapt the original interpretation to the receptor theory, thereby explaining vasomotor reversal by a selective blockade of α-receptors, with the unmasking of the effects which were due to β-receptor activation. The first report on a β-blocker, dichloroisoprenaline (DCI), furnished evidence for this view, since DCI abolished the depressor response to adrenaline observed during adrenergic blockade (Powell and Slater, 1958).

However, no experimental proof was given for the part of this theory, which postulates that before blockade of α-adrenoceptors, adrenaline activates α- and β-receptors and that the hypertensive response represents the algebraic sum of opposing effects on vascular receptors, α-adrenoceptors subserving vasoconstriction and β-receptors inducing vasodilatation (Fig. 1). On the other hand, it has been shown that the long-lasting and unsurmountable adrenergic blockade caused by potent agents such as the β-haloalkylamines Dibenamine and phenoxybenzamine can be

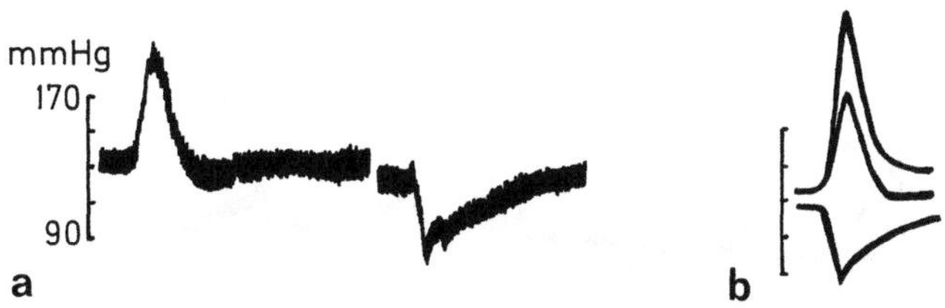

Fig. 1. a Actual blood pressure tracing showing adrenaline reversal in a dog anaesthetized with sodium pentobarbital 30 mg/kg; effects of i.v. adrenaline 2 µg/kg, before and after benzodioxane (883 F) 5 mg/kg i.v. **b** Schematic representation of the unmasking theory of vasomotor reversal. The *upper curve* shows the pressor effect that this dose of adrenaline should exhibit in the presence of a β_2-adrenoceptor blocking agent

New Aspects of the Role of Adrenoceptors in the Cardiovascular System/Ed. by Grobecker et al.

reinforced by ergot alkaloids, benzodioxane compounds or phentolamine (Osswald 1958, 1960). Figure 2 shows a representative example of this phenomenon. The additive effects of adrenoceptor blocking agents were attributed to the existence of receptors not blocked by the β-haloalkylamines, i.e. spare receptors (Osswald 1960). Thus, vasomotor reversal would occur in the face of incomplete α-blockade.

Reversal of Adrenergic Vasodepression: Role of α_2-Adrenoceptors

Another puzzling phenomenon concerns adrenaline "re-reversal", known as reversal of adrenergic vasodepression or negation of α-blockade. Since many α-adrenoceptor blocking drugs show an evanescent effect, it is convenient to limit the discussion to adrenaline re-reversal occurring in animals treated with the "irreversibly" acting β-haloalkylamines. Of the many drugs investigated, only vasopressin, barium chloride and ephedrine consistently caused adrenaline re-reversal in animals treated with phenoxybenzamine or Dibenamine (Ahlquist 1950; Levy and Ahlquist 1957; Maengwyn-Davies and Walz 1958; Osswald 1958, 1960).

Ephedrine was particularly effective in changing the vasodepressor response to adrenaline into a pressor response; this effect appeared to involve a vascular point of action, since intra-arterial adrenaline reacquired, after ephedrine, a vasoconstrictor effect (Levy and Ahlquist 1957; Osswald 1960). It was also clear that the residual pressor response to noradrenaline was potentiated by ephedrine (Fig. 3).

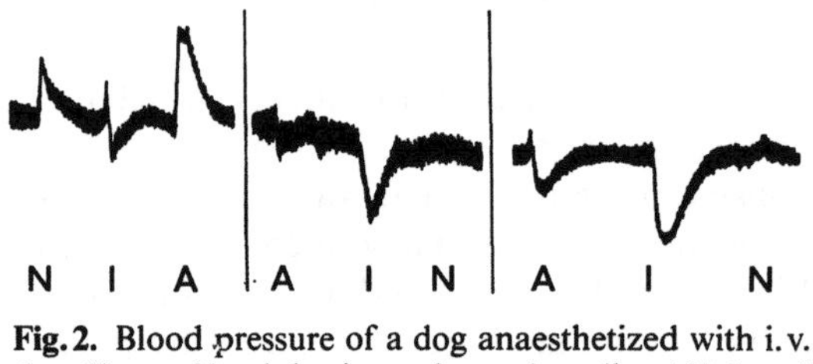

Fig. 2. Blood pressure of a dog anaesthetized with i.v. chloralose (100 mg/kg). The tracing shows the effects of i.v. injections of noradrenaline (*N*, 1 µg/kg), isoprenaline (*I*, 2 µg/kg) and adrenaline (*A*, 2 µg/kg). Between the *first* and the *second panel*, phenoxybenzamine 5 mg/kg was injected; between the *second* and the *third panel*, piperoxan 5 mg/kg was administered

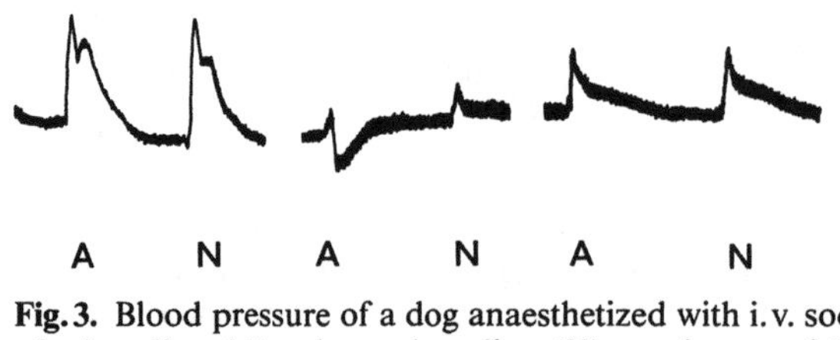

Fig. 3. Blood pressure of a dog anaesthetized with i.v. sodium pentobarbitone (30 mg/kg). Effects of adrenaline *(A)* and noradrenaline *(N)* at a dosage of 2 µg/kg. Between the *first* and the *second tracing*, phenoxybenzamine 5 mg/kg was administered; between the *second* and the *third tracings*, ephedrine 12 mg/kg was given

Some years later, a new type of adrenaline re-reversal was described: β-blockers were shown not only to abolish the depressor response to adrenaline in animals under α-blockade, but were also demonstrated to allow for the manifestation of pressor responses to adrenaline (Hull et al. 1960; Gulati et al. 1965; Moreira and Osswald 1965; Garrett et al. 1966; Olivares et al. 1967; Patil et al. 1968; Yamamura and Horita 1969; Story and Bentley 1974).

Re-reversal was considered as a curiosity in experimental pharmacology, and the explanations offered were many (see Osswald 1960; Story and Bentley 1974). Since the peripheral locus of action of β-blockers has been unequivocally demonstrated (Moreira and Osswald 1965; Garrett et al. 1966; Olivares et al. 1967), two main explanations could be offered: displacement of β-haloalkylamines from α-adrenoceptors (Olivares et al. 1967; Patil et al. 1968) or exposure, by β-blockade, of α-adrenoceptors not occupied by the β-haloalkylamine (Moreira and Osswald 1965; Garrett et al. 1966; Yamamura and Horita 1969). The latter interpretation was based on the following facts: adrenaline never reacquired its full pressor and vasoconstrictor effects, the pressor responses were slower in onset and more prolonged, the dose-response curve was flatter and displaced to the right, and the benzodioxane derivative 883 F abolished these pressor responses to adrenaline (Garrett et al. 1966).

Soon after the existence of postjunctional α_1- and α_2-adrenoceptors in vascular smooth muscle was demonstrated, Constantine et al. (1980) showed that pressor effects of noradrenaline in the dog are mediated by both subtypes of α-adrenoceptors. Confirmatory evidence was provided by the work of other authors (reviewed by Langer and Hicks 1984). In light of this knowledge, Constantine and Lebel (1980) re-examined the adrenaline re-reversal by propranolol in dogs treated with phenoxybenzamine. They found that under these circumstances, α_1- but not α_2-adrenoceptors, were fully blocked by phenoxybenzamine (the residual pressor response to noradrenaline was antagonized by yohimbine, but not by prazosin) and that the pressor response to adrenaline which propranolol caused to reappear (adrenaline re-reversal) was unaffected by prazosin, reduced by corynanthine and eliminated by yohimbine. They concluded that adrenaline re-reversal is explained by activation of α_2-adrenoceptors, thus giving experimental support to the explanation proposed by Garrett et al. (1966).

The re-reversal induced by ephedrine has not been previously explained, and we therefore decided to re-examine this type of re-reversal. Again using pithed dogs treated with phenoxybenzamine, we found that ephedrine (10–20 mg/kg) regularly caused a change in the response to adrenaline, from a purely depressor response to a biphasic or purely pressor effect. In this aspect, ephedrine behaved similarly to propranolol; however, unlike propranolol, ephedrine did not abolish the depressor response to isoprenaline. Thus, it appeared clear that ephedrine and propranolol had different mechanisms of action. This corresponds well to the fact that propranolol and ephedrine had additive effects, i. e. that the hypertension caused by adrenaline in the presence of both drugs was larger than that which was observed after single administration of either of the drugs. Yohimbine (but not prazosin) reduced or abolished the hypertension, caused by adrenaline in the presence of ephedrine; thus, we conclude that this hypertensive response is due to activation of α_2-adrenoceptors. Figure 4 illustrates these points.

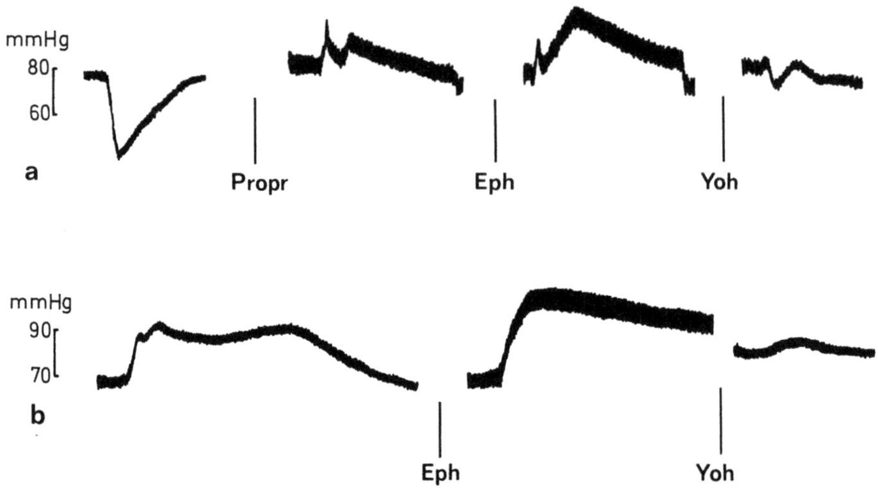

Fig. 4a, b. Blood pressure of a pithed dog injected with phenoxybenzamine 5 mg/kg. **a** Effects of adrenaline 2 μg/kg, under control (phenoxybenzamine) conditions and after propranolol 0.5 mg/kg *(Propr)*, ephedrine 15 mg/kg *(Eph)* and yohimbine 0.2 mg/kg *(Yoh)*. **b** Effects of BHT-920 80 μg/kg, under phenoxybenzamine + propranolol conditions (propranolol did not change the response to BHT-920; not shown), as well as after ephedrine *(Eph)* and yohimbine *(Yoh)*

In a further attempt to define the mechanism of action of ephedrine in inducing re-reversal, we used 2-amino-6-allyl-5,6,7,8-tetrahydro-4*H*-thiazolo-[4,5-*d*]azepine dihydrochloride (BHT 920), a selective α_2-adrenoceptor agonist (Kobinger and Pichler 1980); it was found that the pressor responses to BHT 920, as obtained in the animal treated with phenoxybenzamine, were not significantly affected by propranolol, but were potentiated by ephedrine (Fig. 4).

From these results we conclude that, although both propranolol and ephedrine cause adrenaline re-reversal as a result of activation of α_2-adrenoceptors, the underlying mechanism is different. When α_1-adrenoceptors are blocked by phenoxybenzamine, adrenaline causes a fall in blood pressure because β_2-adrenoceptor-mediated vasodilation prevails. Propranolol eliminates the latter reaction, and activation of the non-blocked α_2-adrenoceptors becomes evident. In the case of ephedrine, although β_2-adrenoceptors are not blocked, the action of adrenaline on α_2-receptors is clearly potentiated and the end result is hypertension.

The Explanation of Adrenergic Reversal and Re-reversal

Our view clearly varies only slightly from the theory proposed so many years ago by Sir Henry Dale, although we attribute reversal not to "unmasking", but rather to a shift in the agonist molecule from receptors occupied by the antagonist to spared receptors. Adrenaline, with its ideal affinities for all types of adrenoceptors, is still an excellent tool for pharmacologists to study the reactivity of adrenoceptors. The blood pressure response gives us important clues about the type of receptors which are activated by adrenaline. We think that under control conditions (and at least for the conventional dose range of 0.5–2 μg/kg) mainly α_1-receptors are acted upon by adrenaline; after blockade of these receptors (by phenoxybenzamine or prazosin), adrenaline molecules are diverted to β_2-adrenoceptors, which they stimulate, and consequently hypotension occurs (adrenaline reversal). If β-receptors are blocked (by pronethalol or propranolol), only α_2-adrenoceptors may still be activated and re-reversal occurs; the same phenomenon is seen when the actions on α_2-adrenoceptors are potentiated by ephedrine. An adequate blocking drug (yohimbine) abolishes these responses. This schematic representation implies different affinities (or accesses) of adrenaline for the different vascular subtypes of adrenoceptors, in the order of $\alpha_1 > \beta_2 > \alpha_2$, with an unknown, although minor, role played by cardiac β_1-adrenoceptors. We are aware that experimental evidence is lacking for this concept, but this proposal best fits the facts so far observed.

Summary

The classical phenomenon of adrenaline reversal is re-examined in light of present knowledge concerning adrenoceptors and their subdivisions. The reversal caused by the long-lasting and "unsurmountable" adrenergic blocking agent phenoxybenzamine in dogs was adopted as a model for this study. It was possible to reinforce the adrenergic blockade induced by phenoxybenzamine by other drugs of the same group (such as the benzodioxane derivatives, yohimbine, ergot alkaloids), but not by prazosin. Thus, phenoxybenzamine appeared to cause complete blockade of α_1-, but not of α_2-adrenoceptors, and reversal occurred when α_2-adrenoceptors were not blocked. On the other hand, propranolol and ephedrine were able to reinstate a pressor response to adrenaline, i.e. to cause "re-reversal"; their effect was additive. Ephedrine, but not propranolol potentiated blood pressure responses to BHT-920, an agonist with selectivity for α_2-adrenoceptors. The pressor responses to adrenaline in animals treated with phenoxybenzamine, propranolol and ephedrine were smaller then those obtained under control conditions. They also showed a different time course and were characterized by a flatter dose-response curve; the pressor responses were abolished by yohimbine.

It is concluded that re-reversal is due to activation of α_2-adrenoceptors and that ephedrine potentiates the effects of adrenaline and BHT-920 on these receptors. Adrenaline reversal is not adequately explained by the "unmasking" theory, but rather by the preferential occupation of different receptors according to the adrenergic blocking drugs which are present.

References

Ahlquist RP (1948) A study of the adrenotropic receptors. Am J Physiol 153: 586–600

Ahlquist RP (1950) Studies on the reversal of epinephrine reversal. J Pharmacol Exp Ther 98: 1

Constantine JW, Lebel W (1980) Complete blockade by phenoxybenzamine of α_1- but not of α_2-vascular receptors in dogs and the effects of propranolol. Naunyn-Schmiedebergs Arch Pharmacol 314: 149–156

Constantine JW, Gunnell D, Weeks RA (1980) α_1- and α_2-Vascular adrenoceptors in the dog. Eur J Pharmacol 66: 281-286
Dale H (1906) On some physiological actions of ergot. J Physiol (Lond) 34: 163-206
Garrett J, Malafaya-Baptista A, Osswald W (1966) Effects of pronethalol on the cardiovascular actions of catecholamines during blockade by phenoxybenzamine. Br J Pharmacol 27: 459-467
Gulati OD, Gokhale SD, Udwadia BP (1965) Antagonism of adrenergic blockade by pronethalol. Arch Int Pharmacodyn 156: 389-397
Hull LD, Eltherington LG, Horita A (1960) The antagonism of adrenergic blockade by dichloroisoproterenol (DCI). Experientia 16: 368-369
Kobinger W, Pichler L (1980) Investigation into different types of post- and presynaptic α-adrenoceptors at cardiovascular sites in rats. Eur J Pharmacol 65: 393-402
Langer SZ, Hicks PE (1984) Alpha-adrenoreceptor subtypes in blood vessels: physiology and pharmacology. J Cardiovasc Pharmacol 6: S547-558
Levy B, Ahlquist RP (1957) Inhibition of the adrenergic depressor response. J Pharmacol Exp Ther 121: 414-420
Maengwyn-Davies GD, Walz DT (1958) Autonomic drugs modifying the effects of N,N-dibenzyl-beta-chlorethylamine (dibenamine) on dihydroxyphenylethanolamines. Arch Int Pharmacodyn Ther 113: 422-426
Moreira JG, Osswald W (1965) Pronethalol-induced reversal of adrenergic vasodepression. Nature 208: 1006-1007
Olivares GJ, Smith NT, Aronow T (1967) Effect of propranolol on alpha adrenergic blockade in the dog and isolated rabbit aortic strip. Br J Pharmacol 30: 240-250
Osswald W (1958) Inversão vasomotora. Thesis, Universidade do Porto
Osswald W (1960) Reversal of adrenergic vasodepression. Arch Int Pharmacodyn Ther 126: 346-358
Patil PN, Tye A, May C, Hetey S, Miyagi S (1968) Steric aspects of adrenergic drugs. XI. Interactions of dibenamine and beta adrenergic blockers. J Pharmacol Exp Ther 163: 309-319
Powell CE, Slater IH (1958) Blocking of inhibitory adrenergic receptors by a dichloro analog of isoproterenol. J Pharmacol Exp Ther 122: 480-488
Story ME, Bentley GA (1974) The effects of drugs and treatments upon adrenaline re-reversal in the rabbit. Arch Int Pharmacodyn 212: 5-23
Yamamura HI, Horita A (1969) A further study of the effect of propranolol on the blockade of alpha adrenergic receptors. Eur J Pharmacol 7: 258-263

Subject Index

MIX
Papier aus verantwortungsvollen Quellen
Paper from responsible sources
FSC® C105338

If you have any concerns about our products,
you can contact us on
ProductSafety@springernature.com

In case Publisher is established outside the EU,
the EU authorized representative is:
Springer Nature Customer Service Center GmbH
Europaplatz 3, 69115 Heidelberg, Germany

Printed by Libri Plureos GmbH
in Hamburg, Germany